I cannot quit thinking about *Aura Personalities*. It is such a blessing in my life, and an answer to a prayer. Thank you so much for your insightful information that helps me to understand myself, and those around me better.
Val Johnston, LCSW
Malad City, ID

Staci Sadler is INSIGHTFUL and full of light. Our family went for an *Aura Personalities* Consultation and it changed two lives. Before the consultation, my 11-year-old son and I were constantly fighting and power struggling. I didn't know how to communicate with him. And he didn't like me very much. When it was his turn to have Staci talk about his Aura colors and personality traits, he lit up. I could tell that her words were lighting a fire in him. They were describing him and he felt a connection with Staci. Later he said, "Mom, when can I go back to talk to Staci? She knows everything about how I think and it feels good to me." Since that first meeting, things have been better between my son and I. If I do not understand where he's coming from, I pick up the *Aura Personalities* book, read through his main aura colors, and it puts me back on track. He has found his wings and is living happier.
Dina Love
American Fork, UT

The *Aura Personalities* book opened my mind up to the fact that we all experience everything differently. Now I am able to more fully teach, be taught by, love and be loved by everyone I know. My relationships have become so much more closely knit. I am truly grateful for this work and I cheer on everyone who participates.
Dallin Hughes
Branson, MO

I love *Aura Personalities*! It has helped me to better understand why I am the way I am and that I don't have to be something different. I have more power to help others now that I can be myself. This knowledge also helped me to better accept and encourage people in who they truly are.
Katie Gamble, LPN, Clinical Research Coordinating Manager
Logan, UT

The whole *Aura Personalities* topic has changed my life and particularly my children's who have participated in aura testing. It brought much needed clarity to our lives and an understanding why we each act and react to people and situations the way we do.

I was very impressed with Staci's ability to *know* me and be so spot on even though she had never met me before. My consultation with Staci was an amazing experience.
Carol Parker, School Administrator
Mesa, AZ

Staci Sadler has an innate gift that reaches into the essence of whomever she communicates with. With this new insight I have since been practicing accepting myself, and allowing myself to dig deeper, and push further the parts of my personality that I thought were weaknesses.
Karla Reyna
Mesa, AZ

Learning about my aura has helped me find peace with how I am different then everyone else. I feel empowered now to be the person I am and I embrace my uniqueness. I am happier then I ever was and feel excited about my future!
Lauren La Rose
Anchorage, AK

Aura Personalities sheds a literal light on the diverse traits and gifts of individuals in the human family. There are many books and schools of thought on personality, but I have found Staci's to go deeper and more thoroughly into the spiritual aspects of inborn attributes and abilities. Her work is truly fascinating!
Cherie Burton, Author & Life Coach
Alpine, UT

In *Aura Personalities*, I found precious treasures regarding who I am, and who others are, and what we each need to respect about ourselves in order to enjoy the fullest happiness possible.
As I learned of different needs of my 3-year-old son, I have adjusted how I interact with him. I understand and can even delight in the way he works and moves, as it is a part of the magnificent being he is and the magnificent work he is here to do. Staci's work has helped me to see his soul, which has changed both of our worlds a million times for the better. Staci's beautiful gift is in seeing who someone really is and helping them and their loved ones develop this precious vision. Since my eyes have been opened through Staci's work, I see my life and all other beings with a refreshing newness, clarity and love.
Natalie Stevens, MFT
Maui, HI

I love this book. I have referred it to many clients and am glad to see their reactions when they figure out who they are and what their potential may be... This book is a great tool to help people find and discover the innate gifts and talents they already have.
Lisa O'Donnal, RN, NAET Practitioner
Lehi, UT

It is not often I come across a truly life-changing book, but *Aura Personalities* has changed my life for the better. It has become an encyclopedia of knowledge for me and my entire family. Staci Sadler's study and description of the human aura, and the personality information therein, is deep and comprehensive. If you have any interest in people and what makes each of us tick, then you will positively devour the information found on these pages. If you have already studied aura colors you will be pleasantly surprised to find the latest research that Staci has tirelessly compiled concerning the "New Crystals."

Staci Sadler is a gifted, caring, and spiritually deep teacher/author/mentor. She is careful to seek out the truth and help her students find their true life-path. This is her passion.
Angie Petersen
Boise, ID

Aura Personalities is an amazing and insightful book. If you have ever desired to understand those in your family, co-workers, friends, and people in general better, this book will open your mind to an entirely fresh and uplifting perspective of everyone around you.
Jennie Ohlund
Cedar Hills, UT

Aura personalities has provided many with a guide to the soul. I am more confident in how I act, I know why I have certain trials, and it has helped me be more accepting of others and how they act. It has opened a window of long forgotten truths that we all once knew and has provided clarity to who I truly am in a world clouded with the judgments of the media and countless others. To me it has been a step towards peace in my life and I share it with all who are ready.
Josh Ohlund
Cedar Hills, UT

After having read *Aura Personalities* numerous times, I've concluded that each chapter has been written with exceptionally clear insight and pure understanding.

Thank you, Staci, for your passion, your time and effort in giving this gift. This amazing book helps the reader to get in touch with the inner self, to a higher degree of understanding, so as to truly walk in harmony with the light of these gifts that are meant to shine and be a blessing to the world.
Tamara Marshall
Boise, ID

Our family had the opportunity to visit with Staci Sadler, Soul Integrity Mentor this past summer. It was a very enlightening experience, both as a parent and as an individual. As we continue to read, and re-*read Aura Personalities*, we not only learn about our true selves, but also about one another, and how to better understand one another.
Celeste Kennard
Frisco, Texas

Understanding *Aura Personalities* is an interesting way to get to know myself and others in my life. Learning from Staci and having some insight of my energy has given me more confidence in my job. It makes me even more aware of the influence I have on people when teaching environmental education.
Kathy Donnell, Park Naturalist
Midway, UT

I was literally awestruck at the amount of 'information' that Staci Sadler was able to assess and/or 'harvest' in less than ten minutes in her presence. I was told that one could learn what she does but she is gifted in other ways as well, particularly in the area of communication and empathy.
Michael Alexander
Idaho Falls, ID

My family owns two *Aura Personalities* books. As a family we have found that knowing our Aura personalities has helped shift the dynamics of our family. We have 9 children and for the first 3 weeks after buying the book…there was at all times a family member on the couch with the book and the list of siblings and their colors. We studied ourselves and each other. The end result is that we have an easier time not taking things so personally…My clients have loved the book as well and it has been a very useful tool in the mentoring and breakthrough process.
Susan Taylor, Owner of Living Equilibrium
Bountiful, UT

Staci Sadler has been gifted with such a beautiful understanding and insight of our auric traits. She has shed Light on aspects of myself I did not understand, or even felt afraid of, that opened my eyes to compassionate insight to myself, and gave me tools to better accentuate my strengths, thus de-emphasizing my weaknesses. This knowledge also helps me to be aware of the ways in which I particularly behave negatively, which knowing that I can better be prepared to choose my Higher ways of being.
Crystal Betterton
Draper, UT

AURA
PERSONALITIES

AURA

PERSONALITIES

OUR INNATE GIFTS & MAGNIFICENT POTENTIAL
REFLECTED IN THE ENERGY WE EMANATE

Staci Sadler

AURA PERSONALITIES. Copyright © 2013 by Staci Sadler. All rights reserved. No part of this book may be used or reproduced in any manner whatsoever without written permission from the author except in the case of brief quotations embodied in critical articles and reviews. For information call (801)477-0714 or email admin@aurapersonalities.com.

Cover photo: Shutterstock leaf image by Sarah Cunningham
Title & Cover Design by Michael Bunn

First paperback edition published May 2012
eBook edition published December 2012
Revised & Updated paperback edition published January 2013

Printed in the United States of America by McNeil Printing

ISBN-10: 1605740187

ISBN-13: 978-1-60574-018-8

www.AuraPersonalities.com

This book is dedicated to Mathias, my little buddy and best teacher, and God, for his daily mercies and boundless love.

CONTENTS

~

To The Reader	3
Love & Gratitude	9
Introduction	11
Muscle Testing	45
The Body Family	57
Green-Amber: *The Naturalist*	60
Yellow: *The Motivator*	71
The Physical-Environment Family	85
Red: *The Landlord*	88
Orange: *The Summiteer*	100
Magenta: *The Creator*	108
The Mental Family	117
Amber: *The Judge*	120
Green: *The Innovator*	132
The Mental-Emotional Family	143
Red-Amber: *The Storyteller*	146
Blue-Amber: *The Ministering Angel*	156
The Emotional Family	169
Blue: *The Heart Guardian*	172
The Emotional-Spiritual Family	185
Violet: *The Influencer*	188

Lavender: *The Free Spirit*	201
The Spiritual Family	215
Crystal: *The Vessel*	218
Indigo: *The Paradigm-Shifter*	228
Aventurine-Crystal: *The Avatar*	243
Magenta-Crystal: *The Saint*	261
Amethyst-Crystal: *The Angel*	278
Indigo-Crystal: *The Commander*	287
Imperial Topaz: *The Phoenix*	300
Shifting Auras	311

TO THE READER
~

The overarching struggle for every person on this planet is the same: To figure out who we are, come to terms with that in the context of this life, and then allow ourselves to shine more fully as the beings of light that we are.

We are each unique in our light. No two people offer the same gifts to the world. In our individuality, however, we also have unique crosses to bear, the things that are most difficult for us and about us. Throughout our lives experiences bump up against these particular traits, magnifying our peculiar tendencies that we call weaknesses.

In one sense, we do have weaknesses and are always capable of inflicting harm due to them, but we also have the strengths to match them, the strengths that are their polar opposites. If you get nothing else from this book, I hope that you will at least begin to see this possibility that at the core of our weaknesses the perfect DNA resides ready to birth our greatest strengths. May you come to view humanity and yourself with more compassion and hope.

The more I have observed and felt the energy and intentions of others, the more certain I am that there is a *Potential Spectrum* within us, at one pole lies our weakness potential, at the other our strength potential. What that means is that we have everything within us to realize greatness.

There is no such thing as just a weakness to extinguish. Weakness exists so that a road exists to travel toward strength. Weakness is not extinguished; it is transformed into strength.

For example, there is a *Potential Spectrum* in a fragile immune system, a specific trait of certain Aura Personalities. On one end of the spectrum reside chronic pain, illness and exhaustion (with its attending wear on the spirit manifesting as depression, hopelessness, a sense of victimhood and powerlessness, and a feeling of separateness from life and other people). These feel very much like weakness to the person who has them. Yet on the other end of the very same spectrum lie gifts that could not be emulated by anyone without those particular weaknesses. These gifts, or strengths include: heightened sensitivity on a sensory level of sight, taste, touch and smell; a first-hand understanding of the body and of our stewardship over our bodies and health, as well as that of others and our planet; true compassion, empathy, a connection and awareness of all suffering; a capability of seeing light and goodness at the core of everyone and everything; a knowledge that power does not come from without, from someone else trying to fix our problems, but comes from within, from our ability to surrender, cope and then let go on a spiritual level to the point that pain can no longer touch us in those infinite places.

From this perspective, a weakness suddenly becomes a pathway to travel to reach our greatest potential, unveiling magnificent gifts that benefit all of humanity. Weakness is the perfect seedling for strength to grow from, once we become aware of it and allow ourselves to consciously learn from it. The only real tragedy happening on our planet at any given time is a person walking directionless, unaware of and imprisoned by such weaknesses when, instead, they could be walking on a transformative path, birthing beautiful strengths from them.

Aura Personalities aims to bring attention to our weaknesses and strengths in the context of the light we emanate. It provides a glimpse into what is possible for all of us if we are willing to see our own light and emanate it with conscious integrity. It is about who we are in the grand scheme of things, even the eternal scheme of things. Habits and traits are included to help us identify our core Aura Personalities but are not its main intention. The main intention is to help us identify and embody the innate gifts and magnificent potential reflected in the energy we emanate.

> *"The soul is dyed the color of its thoughts.*
> *Think only on those things that are in line*
> *with your principles and can bear the light of day.*
> *The content of your character is your choice.*
> *Day by day, what you do is who you become.*
> *Your integrity is your destiny—*
> *it is the light that guides your way."*
> Heraclitus

When we discover the layers of colorful light that surround and emanate from us, revealing our power and our potential, the knowledge can be amazing and feel like true liberation. At the same time, it can also be pretty disconcerting to have sides of ourselves we were happy to keep hidden suddenly acknowledged. But if we are willing to ride through the discomfort, resisting judgment or self-condemnation, keeping our eyes open to the truth, then the journey of self-discovery and emancipation to be who we really are will be astonishing.

Strengths and weaknesses are one-in-the-same at the core, not mutually exclusive. The only way out is in. The only way out of your weaknesses is by going in and seeing the truth about who you are, and that means owning all of the possibilities. You cannot get to your strengths except by traveling honestly through your weaknesses, owning them and then allowing the potential that lies within your light to transform them into powerful strengths.

*Where your weaknesses are,
there will your strengths be also.*

This information is not meant to encourage permissiveness for natural tendencies that are harmful or detrimental to self or others. Rather, it is meant to bring awareness and understanding so our personal stewardships can increase and we can become more fully evolved human beings.

No one came into the world to play small or wallow in darkness. We all came to spread love and shine our unique light. All of us, bar none. In the perfect design of imperfect mortality however, we all forgot our purpose and instead, as Isaiah declared, went astray and *"turned every one to [our] own way."*

Hopefully, understanding our Aura Personalities, will allow us to see what is true about ourselves and turn us back toward God, our light Source. This life really is about remembering who we are and allowing our light to bless others, reconnecting us all to our Source.

> *"A tree forms itself in answer to
> its place and the light."*
> Wendell Berry, Sabbaths 1999 VI

We are light and we are gods in embryo. Our Source is divine so we are divine. When we remember this truth about ourselves and others it is much easier to see that nothing about any of us is a mistake. Nothing about us is an accident. Life is beautifully designed for us to uncover our intricate light. If the Aura Personalities are explored with these principles in mind, the truth about us can launch us into the expansive, God-becoming beings that we are.

∼

AURA PERSONALITIES

LOVE & GRATITUDE
~

This is the kind of book that required collaboration, and love and gratitude are due to many people, those I observed up close, and those I watched from afar for the last several years in order to understand each Aura Personality. Love and gratitude go first to Sheldon and Mathias Sadler, then to Mary Moore and Shannon Hansen for listening directly and indirectly to endless stream-of-conscience thought about what I was intuiting about aura personalities and their attending traits. Thank you to my editor, Stephanie Servoss, for reminding me to trust my voice when writing and relax about the rest. You are hilarious, wise, and a joy to work with. Thank you Rachel Taylor and Cole Bunderson for giving what was needed in editing and support for the first edition, and Natalie Stevens in the second. Love and gratitude to the Albrechtsens, my supportive family-of-origin, for letting me experiment on you and on your children. Your trust in me, even though you were unsure about my methods and this unchartered area called energy work, means the world to me. I extend that trust back to you unreservedly and unconditionally. And finally, the pioneering New Crystals, those I have met and those I have yet to meet, love and gratitude to you for being my teachers and trusting me to introduce your earth-transcending energy to others.

I am an Empath putting to words what I felt around so many people while sharing their energetic space. The more people I meet, the more I sense the immensity and greatness of every soul and am filled with gratitude and reverence for each encounter.

~Staci Sadler

AURA PERSONALITIES

INTRODUCTION TO AURA PERSONALITIES
~

AURA PERSONALITIES

Introduction

THE AURA: BANDS OF COLORFUL LIGHT
Like the atmosphere that envelops our earth, we are each surrounded with a unique atmosphere made up of several bands of different colored light. This rainbow of light is often referred to as the aura.

Each band of light around us signifies certain characteristics about our personalities based on its color. There are up to 19 different colored bands that surround us, but most of us have between 4 and 8 different auric bands. Our combinations of colorful bands make up our unique Aura Personalities.

MAIN AURA PERSONALITY & OVERLAY
The band of light that is closest to and seems to be most integrated with the physical body is called the Main Aura Personality. The color just outside the main color is called the Overlay. Both the Main and Overlay aura colors tell the most about who we are. They reveal characteristics like how we take in information, how we learn, how we communicate, and how and why we

respond the way we do to others and to life. Our Main and Overlay aura colors seem to define how we experience life on a daily basis and over time.

As such, this book will be the most useful if you are able to determine your Main Aura Personality color. A way to discover your Main Aura Personality is to first discover your Main Aura Family.

THE 7 AURA FAMILIES
Each color of light has characteristics that make it part of an Aura Family. Aura colors within the same Family tend to share traits, and they process and interact with life in a similar fashion. The chart below describes the way each Aura Family processes life. To determine which of the 7 families best describes you, ask yourself how you FIRST take in information and what is your FIRST response to any situation. Remember, most of us have between 4 and 8 colors, so we may relate to many of the Aura Families, but identifying the one you instinctively relate to first, will help you identify your Main Aura Personality.

The Aura Personalities are divided into seven families based on the way they process & interact with life, as is demonstrated on THE 7 AURA FAMILIES chart on the following page.

Introduction

THE 7 AURA FAMILIES
How They Process & Interact with Life

AURA FAMILIES	PRIMARY WAY THEY PROCESS & INTERACT WITH LIFE
BODY	With their bodies. Their bodies are their road map through life.
PHYSICAL ENVIRONMENT	In the spatial realm of the physical world. The natural world is a canvas and a school for them.
MENTAL	Through exchange and accumulation of thoughts, information, and ideas. What they know in their minds.
MENTAL-EMOTIONAL	Through interactions, exchanges & experiences with others.
EMOTIONAL	Through their hearts and their emotional connections with others.
EMOTIONAL-SPIRITUAL	Through their emotions, intuition and visions.
SPIRITUAL	Through insight, inner knowing, and spiritual promptings and directives.

HOW DO YOU PROCESS LIFE?

No matter how objective we think we are, all of us are highly subjective. We see the world through a particular lens created by many factors throughout our lives. With figurative blinders narrowing our view, we only see a miniscule part of an infinitely large picture of existence. But if we become aware of our subjective tendencies, the blinders will become more and more transparent.

Understanding our primary mode of operating is a step toward true self-awareness. Instead of something unseen and unknown driving us, we begin to consciously drive ourselves through choices and interactions. Our particular brand of subjectivity, our subjective stance, becomes more obvious and navigable.

We are all responding from a certain energy center FIRST. Identifying our primary energy center (our Main Aura Family) will help us understand our subjective stance. Those energy centers are: the body, the environment, the logical mind, emotion, energy, or a combination of mind and emotion, or emotion and energy. From the following descriptions, you may be able to identify your subjective stance or primary mode of operating and, thus, the Aura Family of your Main Aura Personality:

THE BODY FAMILY: SENSORY

Body Family individuals FIRST process life through their bodily senses. Their subjective stance is sensory. Sensory information is often piggybacked with emotions or thoughts, and can be stimulated by others or the environment. But Body Family individuals experience all of those things first through their bodies—primarily in their torsos and in their muscles, but also through all of their physical senses. The world, others and themselves are defined and understood by their body's sensory reaction to them. These individuals are also fairly practical, literal and straightforward in what they do and do not like. To those who know them well, Body Family people are easy to know and easy to read. They express and show what they are experiencing at any given moment in simple, clear ways.

THE PHYSICAL ENVIRONMENT FAMILY: SPATIAL

Physical Environment Family people FIRST process life by assessing and interacting with their surroundings. They are not person-based but object-based in this way. Their subjective stance is spatial. Physical Environment people are logical and practical, but spatial information is what they use to make decisions. They base much on what they see with their own eyes, hear with their own ears, and learn by their own experience. They do not rely on those outside of them to know what to do or how to be. They are grounded in the present, in reality, but they base their conclusions on the way things have always been done and experienced since the beginning of time. Physical Environment individuals rely on the earth and themselves above all else because both are tried and predictable. They do not feel a need to explain themselves to others. They just do what they are. They wouldn't think of acting any other way. They are not contrived and are very confident-appearing to the rest of us. We always know where we stand with Physical Environment people, and we often rely on them to anchor us in the here-and-now.

THE MENTAL FAMILY: LOGICAL

Mental Family individuals FIRST process life by gathering mental data. Their subjective stance is logical. They will always ask how something makes sense and will ponder a concept until it does, or discard it as useless if it does not. They use previous data to formulate opinions about new data. Their minds are ever engaged in finding conclusions and solutions. You cannot mistake someone in the Mental Family because they are so logical, practical, and unemotional when they speak. They primarily value relationships as a place to exchange ideas and to garner and give respect. There is a sense with Mental Family people that they do not quite believe anything others say, as most of us are not skilled enough to speak as logically and objectively as they value. Most of us are clouded by passion, have a desire for persuasion, or have a personal agenda, whether consciously or not. Mental Family people like facts. Others find themselves repeatedly trying to justify their own positions when really they just need to talk straight and admit when they do not have all the facts. Mental Family people continually want more information about everything, but it is a specific kind of information. They value intellectual, logical and practical material with proven data. With knowledge, these are literal people. They like parameters and platforms, trust research and accumulated data, and build from there. Many of us think we are in the Mental Family because we all learned to communicate, write and deduce based on logic and previous data, but that does not mean it is everyone's FIRST mode of operating. You will know if it is yours because logic and ideas feel like a game, like play. To the

Introduction

rest of us we see the value of logic but find that it does not allow room for full self-expression.

THE MENTAL-EMOTIONAL FAMILY: LOGICAL & EMOTIONAL

Mental-Emotional Family people process life COMBINED, first through their minds and then their hearts. Their subjective stance is logical and emotional. They act from logic and with a plan in mind, and then are persuaded by what their emotions dictate as they carry out their actions. They are offspring of the Mental Family and the Emotional Family, so those in the Mental-Emotional family will find that they highly relate to both.

THE EMOTIONAL FAMILY: EMOTIONAL

Emotional Family people FIRST process life through their feelings, at a fairly deep level. Their subjective stance is emotional. Their intentions and actions nearly always have an emotional foundation. Unfortunately, they do not know how to be true to their emotional selves in a society that values logic, so they often filter their inner-feeling world through logic words in an effort to relate and connect with others. This technique to build relationships often backfires since emotions always find a way to surface. Others feel confused by the mixture of logic words backed by emotional intentions. And the rest of us are unsure and uncomfortable with our emotions, so we resent Emotional Family people for triggering them. But these are the passionate people that dwell in all the emotional extremes of life. They spend the most time in-love as well as heart-broken. They actively campaign for the underdog and any humanitarian causes. They usually use their voice as the instrument to effect change. These are strong individuals, and passion and sentiment are a big part of their strength. We need them to remind us of our hearts and acknowledge our emotions. They give an effective voice to the hearts of us all when they drop pride about appearing too emotional and stop worrying about not being taken seriously.

THE EMOTIONAL-SPIRITUAL FAMILY: EMOTIONAL & TUNED-IN

Emotional-Spiritual Family people process life COMBINED, first through their feelings and then by energetic information. Their subjective stance is emotional and energetically tuned-in. They act with relationships in mind and with a desire to affect individuals or groups on an emotional level. Then they allow unseen information to filter through their highly intuitive minds. Emotional-Spiritual Family people are simultaneously socially interactive while being reflective and private at times. They like learning and honing personal skills while also listening to visions and intuition. They are offspring of the Emotional Family and the Spiritual Family, so those in the Emotional-Spiritual family will find that they highly relate to both.

THE SPIRITUAL (ENERGY) FAMILY: TUNED-IN

Spiritual or Energy Family individuals FIRST process life by how things feel on an energetic level via vibes, nonverbal language, electrical data in their environment, and undercurrents of emotions, agendas and intentions of others. Their subjective stance is energetic. They often feel tapped into a larger agenda, but they do not always know how to name that sensation. Spiritual Family people feel objective in their observations, as do most of the other Families, but they often tune out, in order to "tune in" to wider-ranged and varied frequencies. By

Introduction

doing this, they miss a lot of social connectedness that others enjoy thereby isolating themselves. They often believe they are being ostracized when this happens. Spiritual Family people vacillate rapidly between negative and positive emotions, different levels of energy, and from feeling connected to others and God and then suddenly disconnected from everything, including themselves. Because so much is happening for them internally, they are easily flooded with many kinds of external input. If you have a Main or Overlay in the Spiritual Family, you probably find it difficult to function in many mainstream arenas for long periods.

WAY YOU PROCESS LIFE
From the descriptions above and the seven choices below, try to narrow down the two ways you primarily interact with and process life (your subjective stance or primary mode of operation):

Body Family (Sensory)
Your bodily senses accompanied with emotions and/or thoughts are key _____

Physical Environment Family (Spatial)
You spatially assess and physically interact with your surroundings _____

Mental Family (Logical)
You always gather mental data first in any situation and work on mental problems _____

Mental-Emotional Family (Logical & Emotional)
You act from logic and make a plan, then leave room for emotional responses _____

Emotional Family (Emotional)
Your intentions and actions nearly always have an emotional foundation ____

Emotional-Spiritual Family (Emotional & Tuned-In)
You interact and process with passion and vision but somewhat separately and apart from others ____

Spiritual Family (Energetically Tuned-In)
You read nonverbal cues and sense undercurrents of energy and the agendas and intentions of others ____

LEARNING STYLES
OF THE 7 AURA FAMILES

We learn best when we follow our passions and our interests. Learning is automatic when we desire particular knowledge, and there is always something that our minds, bodies and souls want to learn.

Another way to discern which Aura Family your Main Aura Personality belongs to is to identify your primary learning style. Each of us has a particular way that we learn best and we always focus on the thing that we are most interested in at any given time. Consider WHAT you are most interested in right now and over time. Then ask yourself HOW you learn about that thing. This will help you identify your natural learning style.

Spend some time answering the following questions about your NATURAL INTERESTS and your PRIMARY LEARNING STYLE in the sections below:

Introduction

WHAT ARE YOUR NATURAL INTERESTS?
What do you spend most of your time doing?

What do you spend the most time reading about?

What are you most interested in?

What topics or activities have you been interested throughout your life?

Do you gather information most frequently from the Internet, television, books, conversations, experimentation, or by observation?

Who do you spend the most time with?

What is the content of your interactions with those people?

The above questions should help you know HOW you learn about the things you are most interested in. Based on those responses, how do you learn best?

WHAT IS YOUR PRIMARY LEARNING STYLE?

Mark an X next to each learning technique that applies to you. Also mark an X next to each location that is stimulating for you and fosters learning and growth for you. There should be one family where the learning techniques are most natural for you. Watch for the Aura Families where you have the most X's. Carefully identifying (1) HOW YOU LEARN BEST and (2) WHERE YOU LIKE TO SPEND YOUR TIME can help you know in which Family your Main Aura Personality resides.

THE BODY FAMILY

Learn By:
- __Actively using and paying attention to their senses of sight, taste, touch, smell and sound
- __Using their body to experience new things
- __Being highly physically active on a regular basis
- __Watching cause and effect of their actions on things and on others
- __Traditional school learning combined with a lot of physical activity outside of the classroom
- __Understanding and applying healthy diet principles
- __Understanding and applying health exercise principles
- __Physical competitions of strength, skill or finesse
- __Teamwork revolving around using your body to solve problems
- __Creating art with their hands
- __Conversing while they learn and apply
- __Rehearsing or repetitious practice
- __Experimenting without pressure for a particular outcome
- __Watching demonstrations and then trying them right after or even while observing them

Introduction

__Listening to principles while doing another activity (i.e., knitting, driving, cooking, building, bouncing on a yoga ball, kneading play dough, etc.)

Body Family people might be found learning and applying their knowledge in the following places:

__Environmental venues
__Rehabilitation centers
__Recreational facilities
__Retail stores & venues
__Knocking on doors
__Parties
__Ranches
__Sporting events
__Cruise ships
__Commercials
__Film sets
__Aquariums
__Medical offices
__Sports bars
__Elementary schools
__Junior high schools
__Performance stages

__Health spas
__Health retreats
__Mobile retail
__Assisting roles
__Animal hospitals
__Camps
__Sports teams
__Dance clubs
__Fire departments
__Photo shoots
__Zoos
__Comedy clubs
__Dental offices
__Nursing homes
__Preschools
__High schools
__Social media sites

THE PHYSICAL ENVIRONMENT FAMILY
Learn By:
__Using objects with their body in their surroundings
__Using their practical minds to repair practical materials
__Building, constructing, creating with materials
__Observing how something is done and then trying it, being allowed to practice it whenever they want to and as often as needed
__Figuring it out spatially (anything with parts that need to work together as a whole)

AURA PERSONALITIES

___Figuring things out as they go, not by asking for instructions
___Being able to leave and come back to projects and creations when they are ready to continue without pressure
___Creatively using what is in the environment to meet a need
___Being put into emergency situations where their immediate, impulsive, proactive responses are usually the most helpful for all involved
___Performing or creating on the spot
___Being challenged to exceed or overcome an obstacle or to perform a feat or to beat your last feat or masterpiece
___Moving around while they work or create
___Being able to leave and return to projects
___Having adequate periods to relax and enjoy life intermingled with producing, working and creating

Physical Environment Family people might be found learning and applying their knowledge in the following places:

___Emergency rooms	___Concert halls
___Cathedral walls	___Plantations
___Farms	___Ranches
___Nurseries	___Surgical rooms
___Rehabilitation centers	___Disaster relief sites
___Mountaintops	___Oceans
___Ships	___Rockets
___Railroads	___Prisons
___Rainforests	___Mines
___Police departments	___Fire departments
___Design studios	___Engineering cubicles
___Landscapes	___Production plants

Introduction

__Western films
__Movie sets
__Military regimes
__Gyms
__Construction sites
__Body shops
__Emerging structures
__Emergency response teams
__Action films
__Documentary films
__Olympic stadiums
__Airplanes
__Bridges and dams
__Lumberyards

THE MENTAL FAMILY
Learn By:
__Focusing your mind and filtering out any distractions
__Building ideas from previous ideas to form logical conclusions or to find new solutions
__Fulfilling tasks orderly, one after another
__Setting goals
__Reading any subject that is presented through logic, or where a clear structure and objective are present
__Mental competition
__Peer rivalry
__Debate
__Mental challenges
__Mental puzzles
__Logic games
__Writing about theories and thoughts in order to clarify
__Documenting details and patterns
__Playing with language and linguistics
__Playing with math
__Joining ongoing scientific research
__Philosophizing
__Practicing law
__Practicing rituals and developing precise skills over time and with discipline

AURA PERSONALITIES

Mental Family people might be found learning and applying their knowledge in the following places:

- __Record rooms
- __Laboratories
- __Editors' rooms
- __Courtrooms
- __Crime scenes
- __Hospitals
- __City buildings
- __Electronics stores
- __Historical sites
- __Think tanks
- __Record rooms
- __Peer-reviewed sites
- __Libraries
- __College campuses
- __Law schools
- __Language classes
- __Business offices
- __Computer offices
- __Archeological dig sites
- __Historical Ruins
- __Education Boards
- __Peer-reviewed sites

THE MENTAL-EMOTIONAL FAMILY

Learn By:

__Organizing and planning and then allowing emotions to influence the moment

__A mixture of the Mental Family and Emotional Family modes of learning (combine X's from both lists)

__Choosing a learning method from the "Learn By" section of the Mental Family or Emotional family and then making sure there is an element from the opposite Family always in play throughout the learning and application process

Mental-Emotional Family people might be found learning and applying their knowledge in the following places:

- __School boards
- __Door to door
- __Speaking stages
- __Comedy skits
- __Political campaigns
- __Book clubs
- __Boardrooms
- __Talk shows
- __Television
- __Performances

Introduction

__Business offices
__Classrooms
__Humanitarian centers
__Community programs
__Nursing homes
__Libraries
__Soup kitchens
__Foreign countries

[A good amount of checkmarks in the following 3 Aura Families is probably a good indicator that your Main Aura Personality belongs to the Mental-Emotional Family: Mental Family, Mental-Emotional Family, Emotional Family.]

THE EMOTIONAL FAMILY
Learn By:
__Observing and documenting human interactions and behavior
__Implementing relational principles
__Teaching relational principles
__Listening to and observing others and then paying attention to the feelings in their own hearts
__Thinking about relationships in any setting and asking how are people doing
__Asking others if there is something they can give or do for them to create harmony in relationships
__Partaking of films or books that delve deeply into the emotional and psychological realm of a few main characters
__Making art
__Experiencing dramatic and other arts
__Expressing emotion, passion and great feeling in various modes of art
__Creating harmony between children
__Creating harmony in a family
__Facilitating emotional healing
__Being in a romantic relationship

AURA PERSONALITIES

__Being involved in the details of others' relationships
__Accomplishing personal achievements and going beyond what is expected of them
__Finding ways to surprise people with what they are capable of

Emotional Family people might be found learning and applying their knowledge in the following places:

__Psychology schools __Humanitarian sites
__Disaster relief sites __Art studios
__Art galleries __Welfare offices
__Social work clinics __Reception areas
__Design offices __Preschools
__Therapist offices __Blog websites
__Weddings __Funerals
__Traditional celebrations __Campaigns
__Diplomacy offices __Orphanages
__Birthing centers __Salons
__Spas __Foreign countries
__Hospitals __Medical clinics
__Campuses __Churches
__Schools __Camps
__Career counseling __School offices

THE EMOTIONAL-SPIRITUAL FAMILY

Learn By:

__Acknowledging visions then figuring out how to engage others in them
__Following the thing that interest them the most at any given time and laser-focusing on the part that they are specifically drawn to
__A mixture of the Emotional Family and Spiritual Family modes of learning (combine X's from both lists)

Introduction

__Choosing a learning method from the "Learn By" section of the Emotional Family or Spiritual family and then making sure there is an element from the opposite Family always in play throughout the learning and application process

Emotional-Spiritual Family people might be found learning and applying their knowledge in the following places:

__Schools __Alternative education
__Speaking stages __Performance stages
__Art studios __Design studios
__Music studios __Airplanes
__Office buildings __Reception areas
__Boardrooms __Psychology classes
__Self-help classes __Pressrooms
__Newsrooms __Production plants
__Soapboxes __Campaigns
__Diplomacy offices __Town halls
__Chapels __Sunday school
__Salons __Spas
__Foreign countries __Concerts
__Cruise ships __Courtroom
__Blogspots __Social media sites
__Designing home interiors

[A good amount of checkmarks in the following 3 Aura Families is probably a good indicator that your Main Aura Personality belongs to the Emotional-Spiritual Family: Emotional Family, Emotional-Spiritual Family and Spiritual Family.]

THE SPIRITUAL OR ENERGY FAMILY
Learn By:
- __Inner listening and external observation of what they "hear" from themselves
- __Writing their experience
- __Talking through their experience
- __Making logical sense out of their energy experiences so that others can comprehend them
- __Discussing their thoughts and ideas and experiences freely with peers
- __Having someone listen so they can then listen to themselves and have their ideas evolve
- __Meditating
- __Pondering
- __Using their hands or moving their bodies while they are listening
- __Sitting near the instructor or speaker so that they are within their energy field
- __Sitting in meditative or yoga poses and getting up and moving around whenever they to
- __Being exposed to varied subjects and being able to learn at their own speed, which is very rapid if they are interested in a subject
- __Not being standardized
- __By revealing themselves and what they are learning to others by demonstrating or sharing
- __Having full stewardship over their bodies and minds
- __Being allowed to come and go with any subject, as they are ready
- __Practicing rituals that they are naturally drawn to
- __Observing how people interact and then making decisions about their own behavior based on what they observe
- __Replicating actions of others and the observing their

Introduction

   own reaction to the experience
__Being around people but standing apart and observing
__Practicing polite social behavior
__Unveiling the moral reason behind behavior then adopting the behavior if a good moral reason exists, and likewise ditching a behavior if there is no moral rationale driving it
__Reading novels
__Reading about theories in science and quantum physics
__Being a part of esoteric organizations
__Studying their specific area of interest in-depth until a new one emerges
__Practicing intuition and discernment on a regular basis; ideally, with peers

Spiritual Family people might be found learning and applying their knowledge in the following places:

__Energy centers   __Ancient ruin sites
__Think tanks   __Self-help classes
__Bookstores   __Gaming stores
__Arcades   __Virtual lounges
__Synagogues   __Cathedrals
__Monasteries   __Temples
__Mountains   __Seashores
__Outer space   __Healing rooms
__Nurseries   __Festivals
__Concerts   __Zoos
__Aquariums   __Hospitals
__Rehabilitation clinics   __Space centers
__Holistic health centers   __Engineering cubicles
__Office cubicles   __Classrooms
__Virtual classrooms   __Libraries

DISTINGUISHING THE 19 AURA PERSONALITIES

Each Aura Personality Family contains certain colors. If you are starting to get a sense of which Aura Family you identify with, you are ready to ascertain your Main Aura Personality color. For example, if you seem to process life primarily through your body and its senses, then you belong to the Body Family and your Main Aura Personality is either Green-Amber or Yellow. Or, if you process life through emotions and with visionary ideas, you belong to the Emotional-Spiritual Family and your Main Aura Personality is either Lavender or Violet.

Introduction

THE 19 AURA PERSONALITIES
How They Process & Interact with Life

AURA FAMILIES	AURA PERSONALITIES	PRIMARY WAY THEY PROCESS & INTERACT WITH LIFE
BODY	GREEN-AMBER **NATURALIST** YELLOW **MOTIVATOR**	With their bodies. Their sensory bodies are their road map through life.
PHYSICAL ENVIRONMENT	RED **LANDLORD** ORANGE **SUMMITEER** MAGENTA **CREATOR**	In the spatial realm of the physical world. The natural world is a canvas and a school for them.
MENTAL	AMBER **JUDGE** GREEN **INNOVATOR**	Through exchange and accumulation of thoughts, information, and ideas. What they know in their minds.
MENTAL-EMOTIONAL	RED-AMBER **STORYTELLER** BLUE-AMBER **MINISTERING ANGEL**	Through interactions, exchanges & experiences with others.
EMOTIONAL	BLUE **HEART GUARDIAN**	Through their hearts and their emotional connections with others.
EMOTIONAL-SPIRITUAL	LAVENDER **FREE SPIRIT** VIOLET **INFLUENCER**	Through their emotions, intuition and visions.
SPIRITUAL	CRYSTAL **VESSEL** INDIGO **PARADIGM-SHIFTER** AVENTURINE-CRYSTAL **AVATAR** MAGENTA-CRYSTAL **SAINT** AMETHYST-CRYSTAL **ANGEL** INDIGO-CRYSTAL **COMMANDER** IMPERIAL TOPAZ **PHOENIX**	Through insight, inner knowing, and spiritual promptings and directives.

Although there are similarities between the individual Aura Personalities within each family, there are significant differences as well.

If you are clear on your Aura Family, then distinguishing your Main Aura Personality will be fairly simple because of those differences. The distinctions that help classify each personality are determined, but not limited to the following:

- ❖ MOTIVATIONS
- ❖ PREFERRED STRUCTURES & LIFESTYLES
- ❖ HOW THEY RESPOND
- ❖ WHY THEY RESPOND THE WAY THEY DO
- ❖ LEARNING STYLES
- ❖ INTERESTS
- ❖ PRODUCTIVITY, CREATIVITY, AND WHAT THEY PRODUCE
- ❖ WHAT HINDERS THEM
- ❖ HOW THEY GIVE LOVE AND SUPPORT
- ❖ WHAT SUPPORTS, STRENGTHENS, AND HELPS THEM
- ❖ PRIORITIES
- ❖ VALUES

Introduction

CONSISTENT MODES OF OPERATION

There is some predictability in how we behave or respond to life and to other people. These are called *modes of operation.*

There is nothing hard-and-fast about these categories; they are just general ways the various personalities respond. Note below which of the 3 titles in each box rings true to you, then see if your Main Aura Personality corresponds.

ACTIVE DOERS (Yang Energy)	IN BETWEEN	PASSIVE RECEIVERS (Yin Energy)
Green-Ambers	Yellows	Blues
Reds	Greens	Lavenders
Oranges	Indigos	Crystals
Magentas	Aventurine-Crystals	
Ambers	Magenta-Crystals	
Red-Ambers	Amethyst-Crystals	
Blue-Ambers		
Violets		
Imperial Topazes		

ACTION RISK-TAKERS	VERBAL RISK-TAKERS	EMOTIONAL RISK-TAKERS
Green-Ambers	Red-Ambers	Yellows
Reds	Ambers	Blues
Oranges	Violets	Lavenders
Magentas	Indigos	Crystals
Greens	Aventurine-Crystals	Amethyst-Crystals
Blue-Ambers	Magenta-Crystals	Indigo-Crystals
	Imperial Topazes	

AURA PERSONALITIES

EXTERNAL PROCESSORS	IN BETWEEN	INTERNAL PROCESSORS
Yellows	Ambers	Green-Ambers
Magentas	Blue-Ambers	Reds
Red-Ambers	Violets	Oranges
Blues	Indigos	Greens
Crystals	Aventurine-Crystals	Lavenders
Imperial Topazes	Magenta-Crystals	
	Amethyst-Crystals	
	Indigo-Crystals	

CONCRETE LITERAL THINKERS	IN BETWEEN	ABSTRACT CONCEPTUAL THNKERS
Green-Ambers	Ambers	Magentas
Yellows	Greens	Red-Ambers
Reds	Violets	Lavenders
Oranges	Indigos	Crystals
Blue-Ambers	Magenta-Crystals	Aventurine-Crystals
Blues	Indigo-Crystals	Amethyst-Crystals
		Imperial Topazes

PRACTICAL	LOGICAL	INTUITIVE
Green-Ambers	Ambers	Yellows
Reds	Greens	Magentas
Oranges	Violets	Red-Ambers
Blue-Ambers	Indigos	Blues
		Lavenders
		Crystals
		New Crystals
		Imperial Topazes

Introduction

BLUNT	IN BETWEEN	TACTFUL
Green-Ambers	Yellows	Blue-Ambers
Reds	Magentas	Greens
Oranges	Blues	Lavenders
Indigos	Violets	Amethyst-Crystals
Red-Ambers	Crystals	
Ambers	Aventurine-Crystals	
Magenta-Crystals	Indigo-Crystals	
	Imperial Topazes	

UNSENTIMENTAL	SENTIMENTAL
Green-Ambers	Yellows
Reds	Magentas
Oranges	Red-Ambers
Ambers	Blue-Ambers
Greens	Blues
Crystals	Violets
Indigos	Lavenders
New Crystals	
Imperial Topazes	

NOT PLEASERS	IN BETWEEN	PLEASERS
Reds	Red-Ambers	Green-Ambers
Oranges	Violets	Yellows
Ambers	Aventurine-Crystal	Magentas
Greens	Magenta-Crystal	Blue-Ambers
Indigos	Amethyst-Crystal	Blues
Imperial Topazes	Indigo-Crystals	Lavenders
		Crystals

Hopefully, the steps in this chapter have helped you ascertain at least your Main Aura Personality, if not your Overlay and some of the other Aura Personality layers as well. The last pages of the book contain blank Aura Personalities Charts.

If you are undecided between two colors for your Main Aura Personality, it probably means you have at least discovered your Main and Overlay Aura Personalities but just need to figure out which one you lead with. There are a few things that might help you discern between the two. First, recognize your knee-jerk responses to situations. Second, notice how others respond to you when they first see you, or when you meet someone for the first time. Third, read through the chapters to gain a clear picture of each Aura Personality. Your Main one should become clearer as you filter through the rest.

As you read, you will find that you identify with several Aura Personalities. More than likely, these are the bands of light that make up your complete Aura Personality. Trust yourself and your impressions as you study the chapters. Allow this to be a self-discovery process and an amazing way to understand those around you.

CAUTION IN CATEGORIZING

If you are going through this process for someone else, please keep the following principles in mind:

For many people, being tossed into a category or stereotype is a very stifling experience, one we naturally resist, and for good reason. No one likes to be told they are limited to certain characteristics or behaviors, or that everything they do is a result of a title you have thrown at them. The reason we resist this is because, on some level, we know that we are expansive and limitless in our light and abilities, greater than we would ever suppose.

Introduction

So when you attempt to help someone else understand their Aura Personality, it should never be a source of limiting or trapping them into a category. Narrowing down to a specific Main Aura Personality is offered as a resource for learning about potential and as a way to see the magnificence that already exists in every single one of us.

As you learn the Aura Personalities, please recognize that you are first looking for patterns. So you will naturally draw tight boundaries around your definitions of each personality, distinguishing what does and does not belong to it. As you explore your questions and findings with others, there will be some understandable resistance to what you are sharing. Just have patience. This narrowing and honing in is a necessary and appropriate step in your learning. The more you know, however, the broader your understanding will become of each personality, and the less confining it will feel to others as you share your findings.

Continue on your journey of learning from what is written, but pay attention to your experience around individuals with the particular personalities you are studying. Eventually, you will have a feel for each personality, along with the attending characteristics. On one level, we are knowable, finite beings, but on another level, we are eternal beings aspiring toward infinite potential. If you pay attention you will begin to notice how that infinite potential is unfolding right before our eyes, every moment.

NO ROOM FOR JUDGMENT

There is no such thing as a bad Aura Personality. The worth of all is the same. There is no ascending order. The book simply separates the personalities based on Aura Families, but the order is not ascending. The Body Aura Personalities, defined in the beginning chapters have just as much potential for good as the Spiritual Aura Personalities at the end of the book. Just because someone takes in information "spiritually" does not make them better, just different in how they respond and operate in life. Some Aura Personalities have weaknesses that are more transparent than others, but all the personalities have them. All types of personalities are equally necessary for our planet to progress and fulfill its purpose. All are essential in aiding the rest of us in our journey.

The best part about Aura Personalities is that it helps us dispel judgment of others. The more we learn about the gifts and potential of each individual personality, we can no longer view our way as the only way. Instead, the beauty and generosity in everyone becomes clearer. Everyone is contributing perfectly, just as they are. This does not mean we should not try to improve ourselves. It simply means we are naturally extending light the way we are supposed to, and so is everyone else.

As we become more aware of our light, we can be more purposeful in our radiance. We can own our gifts and use them more exclusively to assist others. And as we become more aware of the light of others, we can encourage them to shine. There is almost nothing in this world like seeing someone for who they are and having them receive acknowledgement from you for it.

Introduction

Amazingly, the light of others instantly shines brighter when it is recognized.

We came here to shine brightly and expel darkness in our wake. So whatever your Aura Personality is, please shine. We need your light.

> *"Let us each take up our flaming torches*
> *and mount as the blazing fireballs of light that we are*
> *and let's burn the sky and leave it with deep scars*
> *and let them be our signatures upon eternity as we go forth!"*
> C. JoyBell C.

~

AURA PERSONALITIES

MUSCLE TESTING AURA PERSONALITIES
~

AURA PERSONALITIES

Several years ago I came across a description of auric energy in a book by Barbara Bowers called *What Color Is Your Aura?*. The author was able to see bands of light radiating from people in an auric field. The colored bands she saw were unchanging in that she was able to distinguish distinct auras around people and somehow describe 14 associated unique personality types. Fascinated with her findings, I wondered if there was a way to know the auric fields of others even if I could not see them. I decided to experiment by muscle testing people to find out their auras.

Auras are light. Light is energy, and energy is electricity. Muscle response testing works because people are electrical conduits. This is clear as we observe how readily lightning uses us as conduits to reach the ground.

OUR BODIES LOVES TRUTH
Muscle response testing is based on the principle that the body cannot lie. The body is energy, as is everything, and resonates and is in constant communication and

interaction with the energy around it. The body is capable of clearly and repeatedly demonstrating that it is physically strong in the presence of truth and physically weak in its absence.

One way to ascertain the strength of the body is to have an individual extend their arm laterally, parallel to the ground, and keep it in the air. Another individual makes a statement and then pushes down on that extended arm with their hand or fingers while the test subject tries to keep the arm up. The arm will stay up if the statement is true, but will drop down if the statement is false, no matter how hard the person tries to keep it up.

Our bodies have innate integrity and can only show a strong muscle test for things that already exist. Alternately, the body cannot give information about things that do not yet exist.

A lie detector operates through the same principle: The person is an electrical conduit sitting in a chair with their feet on the ground. They are connected at the wrist with a wire to a computer, which is connected to an outlet that is electrically grounded. Connected they create a closed circuit.

A lie detector test shows a loss of energy in the body of the person when they lie but no change of energy when they tell the truth. A lie detector test demonstrates that we are physically weakened when we lie.

There are probably unlimited ways to create a closed electrical circuit with the body besides extending the arm and applying pressure. The tester just needs to tell the body the parameters of the test with words and a clear intention, and create a closed circuit. When the tester makes clear, known statements, the body can confirm those statements by holding strong, or not confirm them by being unable to stay strong (or not being able to keep the circuit closed).

MUSCLE-TESTING AURA PERSONALITIES

It took some time to learn to muscle test the Aura Personalities consistently and clearly, much more time than other things I have tested over the years. But it eventually came. What I have found in my experimenting with muscle testing is that if I am calm, present and detached to any particular outcome as the tester, then the person's Aura Personality is made known by a clear, strong muscle test. In those cases, the room feels peaceful and the test is clear to both the tester and the person tested.

The light we radiate is clear and knowable. It is not a secret and is even visible to some. We are emanating it all of the time—influencing, affecting and being affected by everyone and everything around us. Muscle testing is just a way to name what is already known about a person's light.

My knowledge and/or intuition may tell me the colors of light around a person, but a muscle test allows their body to confirm what is known more absolutely. I personally prefer that clarity and objectivity. It allows me an opportunity to stay one step away from something that is very personal and revealing for the person tested. What is tested is about them and for them. I am simply someone who pushed on their arm so their body could confirm the colors of light they emanate. I prefer the neutral role that muscle testing (as a means of ascertaining Aura Personalities) allows. What they do with the information is up to them.

MY JOURNEY INTO AURAS

As I first muscle tested Aura Personalities, I explained auras to people based on what I learned from Barbara Bowers' book, but as I continued to tell people about themselves, I realized I was providing additional and different information coming to my mind intuitively and instantaneously as I spoke. Once I realized what was happening, I made a conscious effort not to learn about auras from any other source, including *What Color Is Your Aura?,* in order to annotate what I was gathering about each personality on my own. I also found I needed to expand upon the aura families. As this intuitive information grew, people wanted access to study it and pass it on to others and thus *Aura Personalities* as a book was born.

NEW CRYSTALS

Early on in my testing of auras I came across many children, and a few adults, whose personalities were unknown. I proceeded to use muscle testing to see if they had new aura colors. In doing so, I found three previously unidentified Aura Personalities, all within the Spiritual Family. For the last few years I generically labeled them New Spirituals 1, 2 & 3. Then, days before sending the first edition of this book to print, in a collaborative effort, we found the color of light associated with each. New Spiritual 1 is Aventurine-Crystal, New Spiritual 2 is Magenta-Crystal, and New Spiritual 3 is Amethyst-Crystal. Just before printing the second edition, two additional Aura Personalities were identified: another New Crystal called Indigo-Crystal (a very cool, light blue color washed through iridescent crystal light), and Imperial Topaz (a brownish, tannish, yellowish light). Indigo-Crystal is a fairly new light around people whereas Imperial Topaz has always been here, just in very small numbers. But that seems to be changing.

ROOM FOR ERROR & MORE DATA
At the time of the second printing, there are a total of 19 Aura Personalities. Please note the possibility for error and the limitations of people, myself included, in making statements for the body to confirm with muscle tests. After all, how can we ever be sure we are following the correct line of questioning? After all, some of my paradigms about Aura Personalities have shifted even since the first edition of this book. The reason I push forward with the information I receive, despite potential contradictions and unexpected blind spots, is because it continues to unfold. It builds upon itself and the blind spots are eventually replaced with more truth about auric light.

I have written and expounded about Aura Personalities in conjunction with muscle testing because of my own experience with the information and how much it has helped me in my own life, but even more so because of the empowerment I have watched it awaken in the lives of so many others over the years. That said, I do not think I am on the only path of truth about Aura Personalities, but I am on a path that keeps opening up before me.

Aura Personalities may be one small way to view our experience in this world. It may be a way for some of us, even if just for a brief moment, to make sense of life and others. It may even serve some larger purpose on a grander scale to which we have no privy to view at this time. Whatever the larger purpose, I do believe many of us are seeking a connection to the Divine, the Source of all Light and Truth, by examining the light we emanate. By identifying the unique light that surrounds each of us, our connection to that Source certainly brightens and expands.

From my experience with it thus far, Aura Personality information and the questions it triggers are like iridescent shafts of light, drifting and changing with each day and each season. There is no such thing as pinning down light; of that I am certain. It is in continual motion—expanding, blending, illuminating. I love that. For that reason I remain unattached to any of what I write in this book, and suggest the same to those who learn it. We cannot lose connection to the wonder of the Universe in our anxiousness to define. Aura Personalities are rays of light that emanate from us, but light is not to be confined, and it can probably never be fully known or defined. It is a magnificent and trustworthy teacher however, so let it take you where it will. Let it open you in ways you are ready to open. Allow yourself to experience a broader expanse of what makes up you. Then keep the door open because we are only on the precipice of a vast universe of truth about the dimensions of light and the Source of all Light.

WORK-IN-PROGRESS
This book is definitely a work-in-progress. Each time I share with others about their Aura Personalities, new bits of information come through as I speak. Due to the nature of this information, I would never be able to

finish writing a book about Aura Personalities because who is to say when the final word will come. Claiming access to such information, I know I am not the only person with this ability, but I do feel accountable for what I personally have received, and feel a strong stewardship over what has come through me up to this point. I know more will come because it has been ongoing since the moment I opened myself to this work.

My intentions in receiving the information and sharing it are spiritual in nature. They are not to point out specific career paths for individuals or create perfect love matches but, instead, are meant to serve as spiritual compasses for those wanting to better understand their own souls so they can shine in radiance and take accountability for the extension of their gifts and talents. I hope you can read it in that same spirit in order to see some truths about who you are and why you are part of this human family at this particular time on our beloved planet.

TRUTHS ABOUT YOUR LIGHT

All aura colors sit somewhere along the electromagnetic spectrum. Crystals and New-Crystals are blended light. Crystal auras look like white light with bits of all the other colors scattered throughout. The best word to describe it is opalescent. New-Crystals are the same as Crystals but the white light is washed with their respective hues. All visible colors of light combined make white light.

WE EMANATE LIGHT

Your Aura Personality is unique to you. It is light emanating from the core of your physical body and extending well beyond it. Some people are able to see colorful light around others; most of us are not. Most people who see auras with their eyes are generally witnessing what is going on with others in that moment. The energy or light they perceive is circumstantial and impermanent, albeit valuable information. The auric light referred to in this book, on the other hand, is something else. It is a continual stream of information communicated to the world through your energy field. It consists of layers of energy, or light, emanating from your whole being all of the time, without you doing anything to make it so. Aura Personalities are amazing because they are so expansive. The bits of light that make up our auras continually reveal truths about who we are.

Your aura is not circumstantial. It tells about who you really are, and it is telling it all of the time. Each bit of light you emanate is a particle of spiritual DNA revealing what is true about you and your purpose here on earth. It is your personality at the core with all of its ramifications, and it is unique to you. No two people are exactly alike, so there is no one exuding light and giving love exactly the way you do.

You are extending yourself out into the world all of the time with your particular light show. All you had to do for this was show up at your birth. But something inside of you and all of us is dissatisfied with just showing up. Just as light is unsatisfied with being contained, so are we. We are meant to emanate and radiate, expand and enlighten. This is the nature of light, and we are light. If you will take the time to see yourself in all your weaknesses and your strengths, you will be astounded by your own magnificence. You will know more surely that you are truly offspring of God, the Source of all Light.

> *"[God] said that we were "gods"*
> *and He is going to make good His words.*
> *If we let Him…He will make the feeblest*
> *and filthiest of us into a god or goddess,*
> *dazzling, radiant, immortal creature,*
> *pulsating all through with such energy*
> *and joy and wisdom and love*
> *as we cannot now imagine…"*
> From *Mere Christianity*, by C.S. Lewis

~

AURA PERSONALITIES

THE BODY FAMILY

~

AURA PERSONALITIES

The Body Aura Personalities

The Body Aura Personalities experience life primarily through their bodies. Their first reaction, response or instinct about anything is sensory. They trust their gut above all else. The body is their great teacher about life and other people and, if they move their bodies while they learn, the Body Aura Personalities can assimilate almost any information.

These kinesthetic learners have the constant belief that things are fine and that everything will be okay. Just being in their presence provides an underlying sense of optimism and peace. The Body Aura Personalities are blessed with the gift of hope, and that, in turn, is the gift they offer to the rest of us.

Theirs may seem a simplistic or naïve way of life, but their innate ability to accept life is a better anecdote for fear, trial or sorrow than almost anything else. Be grateful for the hope that stands next to you in your family or place of work, and never underestimate the value of their easygoing constancy.

The Body Aura Personalities are:

GREEN-AMBERS
YELLOWS

~

THE GREEN-AMBER AURA PERSONALITY

The Naturalist

"Stately and tall he moves in the hall,
The chief of a thousand for grace."
From *Life of Olympus*,
By Kate Franklin

THE NATURALISTS
Green-Ambers are The Naturalists of the Aura Personalities—at one with the environment and with the land. They are instinctive and at home in nature; confident and comfortable with animals; at peace in their own skin; and able to take full advantage of the joy that comes from having a body.

Green Amber ◆ THE NATURALIST

> *"The natural is so awesome
> that we need not go beyond it."*
> Ruth Hurmence Green

Time alone in nature is one of the best ways for Green-Ambers to maintain a sense of self and stay connected to the natural rhythms of life. Nature provides all that they need and they enjoy the challenge of utilizing the power of nature in that way. Green-Ambers demonstrate how to be at ease in solitude. They are like a warm, gentle wind in the desert, naturally making their mark but leaving everything in harmony, just as they found it.

> *"It is of practical value to learn to like yourself.
> Since you must spend so much time with yourself
> you might as well get some satisfaction out of the relationship."*
> Norman Vincent Peale

GRACEFUL & STRONG

Green-Ambers are like horses and deer. They are beautiful, graceful, independent, confident, instinctive and sturdy. They have strong physical constitutions and athletic grace. Although they can be found participating in competitive team sports, they are more often involved in individual physical training. Green-Ambers gravitate toward dance, martial arts, fencing and anything else where discipline, endurance, and artistry with the body are involved. Even their voices can have a rich resonance that is grounding and soothing to hear. Their bodies are their instruments in every way.

BODY CONFIDENT & REGAL

Green-Ambers have unparalleled, innate body confidence. They exude confidence as they carry themselves gracefully through life; the fact that they are not conscious of their grace just enhances it. Green-Ambers just look royal and untouchable. This is not something to be learned, it is just one of the gifts of their energy field.

> *"Grace is beauty in motion."*
> Henri Fuseli

Green-Ambers move with such unconscious harmony and grace that the rest of us cannot resist watching them. They are the timeless beauties of this world with visual harmony in feature and expression. Green-Amber men might be uncomfortable being called beautiful, but the harmony of their form and the way they move cannot be called anything less.

QUIET & UNAPPROACHABLE
Green-Ambers have naturally reposed facial expressions that imbue them with a distant, mysterious air. It usually takes one conversation to dispel their mystery. People are always pleasantly surprised with how mild and kind Green-Ambers are once they speak with them.

PURSUED OR REJECTED FOR APPEARANCE
Our own insecurities are what get in the way of relationships with Green-Ambers. They did not choose to have everyone respond to them based first on their appearance. Many of us do not make the effort to get to know Green-Ambers and choose to remain intimidated or threatened by their stately demeanor.

Those that do befriend them often have ulterior motives. They befriend them because they are attractive, or pursue them out of curiosity, a strong attraction, or a desire to win them, rather than wanting to truly know them. For this reason, Green-Ambers often feel lonely and separate, unsure of the motives of others, fearful to breach the invisible barrier between themselves and everyone else. This is especially true for women, but Green-Amber men also feel socially isolated at times.

Those who love the challenge of the chase, spend a lot of energy and resources to catch Green-Ambers. Once conquered, however, they quickly learn that they have projected the deep mystery and continual challenge onto Green-Ambers and often discard them for a newer model or bigger challenges.

EASY—GOING & AUTHENTIC
Despite appearances, Green-Ambers are easily won, especially if their gut tells them it is okay to go ahead with the relationship. In fact, Green-Ambers accept and trust others easily and are generally easy-going people.

Green-Ambers are true to themselves and true to their interests. People and relationships are the only area that gets fuzzy for them because they really want to trust. However, they are clear about whether or not they are interested in others. They either approve of you or not and, if they do not, they will not pretend to. But, despite their standoffish demeanor, they are not a hard sell. If there gut tells them to go ahead with a relationship, they will. They actually accept most people quite easily.

PRACTICAL & BLUNT
Green-Ambers are not eloquent in speech. They say what is on their mind and often speak without thinking. They do not see the need to beat around the bush, so they speak bluntly in order to get to the point, harsh or not. They can be quite oblivious of the effect their words

have on others and are sorry when they find they have offended someone.

Green-Ambers are practical in their approach to life and have a hard time relating to those who approach life from a different angle. To be understood by them, the best approach is straight-talk. Green-Ambers respond to bluntness and that is why they dish it out to others.

Green-Ambers are highly capable with tasks and expect the same of others. They assume others can do things more simply and efficiently and can get in trouble with their words when speaking about those topics. What they need to realize is that some of us have much more complex systems—mentally, emotionally, and energetically—and, therefore inhabit more intricate lives than Green-Ambers. Their simplicity is great, but it is important for them to understand that it is not the best kind of life for everyone.

WHAT YOU SEE IS WHAT YOU GET

Green-Ambers are what they are, and they are very straightforward in who they are. They are lovely, uncomplicated, simple, sound and stable, and they are truly the easiest of all the personalities to understand. They are not hiding anything and they even like being known.

Green-Ambers are not center-of-attention people. They are introverted and understandably hesitant in approaching others, but still friendly and sociable when approached. They have a light touch and do not impose themselves on others. They enjoy the company of others but have no problem being alone.

SIMPLE & ACCEPTING
They are simple and practical in the way they think and operate. It's not that they are simpletons; it is just that they do not complicate or fester over things they cannot change. They have the gift of letting things go. They do not waste energy or resources on things that are not useful or practical in some way.

Green-Ambers do worry—but it is more of a fretting over daily tasks and events than a deeper anxiety. They are too present in their bodies to be overly concerned about the past or the future. They generally accept life and events as they are and go with the flow. Overall, Green-Ambers trust the process of life and maintain a sense of acceptance and peace throughout their lives.

As parents, Green-Ambers are nonintrusive and easy going. They are essentially unaffected by the noise and chaos that children bring. They are not easily ruffled and can take things in stride. Green-Amber women have bodies that are custom-made for carrying and bearing children, and both genders have the physical stamina it takes to care for and carry out the tasks and responsibilities of family life. And they enjoy the clarity and simplicity of domestic roles.

CRAFTSMEN & WOMEN
Green-Ambers are good with their hands and strong. They beautify their surroundings with their labors, making everything simultaneously more aesthetically pleasing and more useful.

RESOURCEFUL HOMEMAKERS
They are efficient, practical and unsentimental and can create comfort and a sense of home with very little

material means. They make do with what they have been given. They share this trait with Reds.

Green-Ambers bring the peace and acceptance they generally feel within themselves into their environment. They turn places to live into homes and function very naturally in the role of homemaker. They enjoy the tasks and projects required to run a home—gardening, cooking, raising children and following a routine.

GENTLE STEWARDS OF THE LAND
They are gentle stewards of the land. Their imprint on nature is light because of their innate understanding of man's place in nature. They respect natural laws and are obedient to them. They are like Adam and Eve, tending the garden, multiplying and replenishing the earth, at peace in the world that God has made for them. They are tireless and productive in their labors, able to find joy in the simple tasks and events of life.

Green-Ambers are at peace with themselves and with life and, if you are kind to them, they will be at peace with you and bring you a sense of peace in your life.

PASSIVE & PLEASERS
Because Green-Ambers take so readily to tasks, too many tasks might be left to them. They are pleasers and love feeling a sense of belonging and acceptance. They do not ask much of others and generally let the other person lead in their relationships. Green-Ambers minimize issues and turmoil in their own and others' lives in an effort to maintain peace. They say things are no big deal to avoid conflict. This can be frustrating for those closest to them when something is a big deal. Do not assume, however, that their lack of enthusiasm

surrounding problems means they do not care because they do. They only know how to express things in simple terms without a lot of fanfare. Green-Ambers cope with stress by bottling it up inside, getting anxiety knots in their stomachs, just like Yellows. However, Green-Ambers release this built up stress by moving their bodies. Exercise is a very powerful way for them to emotionally detoxify.

KNOW ABOUT LIFE THROUGH THEIR BODIES

Green-Amber bodies function like sonars. They know about others and things in life via how it relates to their bodies, through their physical senses. Like Yellows, they know and experience the world through their solar plexus, but Green-Ambers have more overall body sensitivity than Yellows. Their bodies are instruments for reading people and making sense of outside stimuli and information.

STEWARDS OF THE BODY

With such fine-tuned physical senses, Green-Ambers are the True North for body care. They know instinctively how to best care for the body and be responsible to it. They watch the body closely, take great care of it, and give it great value. Their attention and awareness of the physical body—on every level and in every aspect—surpasses that of any other personality. They are often drawn to fields that allow them to use their bodies and learn about the body as a whole. These fields include working with animals, acting, modeling, sports, military service, medicine, health, exercise and nutrition.

APPEARANCE-MOTIVATED

They tend to talk a lot about appearance and others tend to bring it up around them often. We all think about our own appearance more around Green-Ambers. The heightened sensory input Green-Ambers experience, coupled with the attention they receive from others for their appearance can create an unhealthy over-focus on the body. Body image and eating disorders are not uncommon for them, especially in their teenage developmental years.

HEALTH ADVOCATES & PROMOTERS

Although it can be tiresome for Green-Ambers to have others focus so much on their bodies and appearance, it is actually where one of their greatest gifts lie. In many ways, no one has more information about the physical body than Green-Ambers. They are the spokespeople for health and exercise because they so naturally live it. They are obedient to what the body needs. They demonstrate healthy behaviors at very young ages. They seem to just know how to relieve stress from the body, they understand the importance of regular sleep patterns, and they are drawn to healthier food with the desire and discipline to eat well and exercise regularly.

OBEDIENT TO NATURE

Green-Ambers are tapped into the natural rhythms and instincts of nature. They have those instincts for health and survival that we see most clearly in the animal kingdom. They can lose touch with those instincts for many years but generally reconnect with it in early adulthood. When they do reconnect, watch out, because they jump into health full throttle. They learn about healthy food and lifestyles and immediately incorporate the principles into their daily lives.

Green-Ambers are very naturally disciplined in their bodies and overall health. Because of this, they are some of the best teachers of health, nutrition and exercise. Their whole appearance is a walking billboard for health principles. We cannot help but want to know what they know and do what they do to have even a small portion of the beauty, strength and vigor they inhabit.

EXEMPLIFY BODY INTEGRITY
Green-Ambers have the true grace of Nature woven into their beings. Others are attractive, but Green-Ambers encompass beauty and functionality as an integrated whole.

These beautiful creatures have true body integrity and have so much to teach us about living in harmony with our bodies. They teach us accountability for our health. They are synchronized with nature and are the aura personality with the most innate obedience. They teach us, by example, to find satisfaction and acceptance in the mundane labors of home and life. When they learn something, they incorporate it immediately into their lives. They are disciplined, instinctive and unquestioning in life.

If we can get over the insecurities these regal beings invoke in us, we might grasp at least a part of the many lessons they have to teach us about living in peace and harmony in this world and in our bodies.

GREEN-AMBER FAMOUS PEOPLE*
Jacqueline Kennedy Onassis (Blue)—former U.S. first lady, art/historical preservationist and fashion icon
Reese Witherspoon—actor
Elijah Wood (Aventurine-Crystal)—actor
Robert Pattinson (Blue-Amber)—actor
Zac Efron—actor, dancer and singer

AURA PERSONALITIES

Rob Lowe—actor
Jennifer Lopez—actor, dancer and singer
Audrey Hepburn (Violet)—actor and UNICEF ambassador
Julia Roberts (Violet)—actor
Catherine Zeta-Jones (Violet)—actor
Cindy Crawford—model
Tyra Banks (Lavender)—model and talk show host
Heidi Klum—model, fashion designer and producer
David Beckham—athlete and UNICEF Goodwill ambassador

*Parentheses signify the secondary part of their main Aura Personality.

~

THE YELLOW AURA PERSONALITY

The Motivator

"Whatever else history may say about me when I'm gone, I hope it will record that I appealed to your best hopes, not your worst fears; to your confidence rather than your doubts. My dream is that you will travel the road ahead with liberty's lamp guiding your steps and opportunity's arm steadying your way."
Ronald Reagan, 1992

SUNSHINE
Yellows are like the sun, radiating warmth to others from their whole being. They shine all of the time, except when they are momentarily eclipsed by sadness,

disappointment or frustration—their own or someone else's. Like a stray cloud moving across the face the sun, the gloomy mood of a Yellow passes as quickly as it comes. In fact, they can be called dispersers of rainclouds for the rest of us. With their genuine, lighthearted nature, and natural ability to let go of hurt or angry feelings once expressed, it is difficult to maintain a low mood in their presence.

EMOTIONS ON THE SURFACE
Like children, Yellows are close to the source of their emotions. They could not hide them, nor would they think to. The emotions of Yellows, whatever they might be at any given moment, are right on the surface, easily expressed and easily read. Everyone knows exactly how Yellows feel at any given time. They manifest emotions clearly and without guile. Yellows do not harbor hidden agendas or ulterior motives. They are who they are, and it is as obvious as the weather.

EMOTIONALLY TRANSPARANT
Others might call them moody, but really they are just refreshingly transparent with their feelings, even as adults. If they visit sorrow, they do not tarry long. Walking through the emotional upset of a Yellow is like walking through a spring shower. It cleanses and suffices the sad heart, and then the sun is suddenly shining once again.

*"All the actions and attitudes of children
are the luxuriant and immediate offspring of the moment,
vested of affectation and free from all pretense."*
Henry Fuseli

Yellow ✦ THE MOTIVATOR

TENDER-HEARTED & FORGIVING
Yellows are tenderhearted, kind, and as vulnerable and forgiving as children. They do not hold grudges for long because it requires too much negative energy—and negative energy just does not stick to them.

LIVE FULLY IN THE MOMENT
Yellows are refreshing to be around because they live in the moment. They do not dwell in the past or hang out in misery, nor do they allow themselves to be encumbered by overly analytical thoughts. There is no one like a Yellow to bring you to the activity of the present. They are engaging and live to interact.

PHYSICALLY ENERGETIC
Yellows are generators of energy and activity. They inhabit Newton's Law that a body in motion tends to stay in motion and, man, are Yellows in motion!

All their lives Yellows are told to: sit still, keep your hands to yourself, stop kicking the seat, give me some space, stay in your chair, and stop wiggling! Stop, stop, stop is what they repeatedly hear. In a way, they are being told that inhabiting, moving and enjoying their bodies is wrong.

MOTIVATORS
Yellow personality gifts lie in their energy and their ability to harness that energy to motivate the rest of us. They are the catalyst to get the rest of us in motion when we are stuck physically, emotionally, or in our beliefs. A Yellow can shake you right out of a funk. Like children their message is: "wake up, it's time to play." They bring us into the moment and help us enjoy today. They remind us to feel joy in using our bodies. Yellows

effortlessly teach joy because they are the embodiment of joy.

> *"Live, love, laugh, leave a legacy."*
> Stephen R. Covey

TRUSTING & GULLIBLE

Yellows are extremely social and can chat it up with the best of them. They are naturally trusting and gullible, but only to a point—they can and will get you back; they like that kind of banter, joking and social interplay.

Yellows understand and love tinkering with social rules. They set the standard for "cool." They have an innate understanding of what is hip in fashion and mores, and what is not. And, through their behavior they keep the rest of us current.

Yellows are not chipper, chirpy birds or irritatingly sweet. Not at all. They are just cool, social and always know where the party is. And when you are around them, you get the sense that you and the world are a little more okay than you previously thought.

ABILITY TO BEFRIEND ANYONE

Yellows have plenty of friends and love friendship. They are fearless with people and will talk to anyone. Deep down they assume everyone would want to be their friend. This comes from a core belief that everyone is worthy of friendship, as well as their innate ability to befriend anyone. Being married to a Yellow is like being married to your best childhood playmate.

SOCIALLY INTERACTIVE

They key with Yellows is interaction. If they are interacting, they are happy. And they are happy interacting because they feel useful. It is in interaction that their gifts can be fully manifest.

CURIOUS EXPLORERS
Where Greens can never have enough ideas to think on, Yellows are incessantly curious. In a Curious George sort of way, they want to explore, taste, touch, climb on, and test out everything they come across. They will try almost anything once. They research and experiment with their whole bodies. Where most of us stop using all of our senses once we learn to speak, Yellows continue exploring the world on a multi-sensory level for their entire lives.

KINESTHETIC LEARNERS & DEMONSTRATORS
Yellows learn and teach others very effectively in this sensory-experiential way. They are kinesthetic learners: they observe and then do. They need to talk about and demonstrate what they learn immediately. This is how they learn. They are often diagnosed with ADHD when really they are just people gifted in kinesthetic language, like their Green-Amber relatives.

Many learning opportunities are missed with Yellows when they are expected to sit quietly and listen. Being expected to read and memorize while sitting still, like many curriculums require, is very taxing on them. Because of this disconnect in the education system with kinesthetic learners, Yellows can go either way: Curious Learners or Distracted Disrupters.

Yellows like attention because they need interaction. For this reason, they can be interrupters because they will take negative attention over no attention. They are often class clowns, performers and pranksters, but their pranks are often light-hearted, and meant to entertain.

ENGAGING & INTERACTIVE TEACHERS

Yellows learn by watching and then mimicking what they see, but an ideal learning environment for them also includes plenty of room for questions and interaction. Talking and moving are how Yellows integrate knowledge. Yellows are natural teachers in this kind of free-flowing learning environment as well.

Yellows become fascinated and completely engaged when learning about something they are interested. They tend to binge on subjects and then quite naturally and enthusiastically share their knowledge with others. It is like they cannot help themselves. They get absorbed and become what they are learning. That demeanor is quite remarkable and their passion quite endearing. It really helps students open up to what Yellows have to teach.

Yellows teach by demonstrating for and interacting with their students. They are very flexible, enjoyable and engaging teachers. Play and relaxation are brought into whatever they teach. It brings Yellows great pleasure to help others learn things that they are passionate about. There is not a lot of ego involved when Yellows are teaching; they just want to share their joy and enthusiasm to enrich the lives of others.

> *"Stay committed to your decisions,
> but stay flexible in your approach."*
> Anthony Robbins

TEACHING US THAT MOVEMENT IS HEALTHY

Imagine for a moment, that we allowed movement in our learning, that it was socially acceptable to shift positions, or get up and walk around, or speak right in that moment when expressing our thoughts to someone else would help us break through to a core concept. It would certainly look different, but there is no reason that order and natural expression could not coexist in the classroom. In fact, if movement were allowed in the classroom, our physical and emotional health would immediately improve, and grades would probably follow.

CENTER-STAGE PERFORMERS

Because Yellows are so sensory and kinesthetic, the dramatic arts can be a very effective way for them to express themselves, as well as demonstrate knowledge learned. They often use their bodies as part of the way they interact with and entertain others. The stage is a natural place for them to "shine" as the center-of-the-sky that they are. But any kind of showmanship will do: sports, creativity, leadership, or sales. Give them an arena to shine in, and they will light it up.

Yellows also have another performance ability that they learn quite young. Yellows know how to appear calm, cool and collected on the outside regardless of what is going on inside of them. They have a tendency to master the tough exterior better than anyone because they are uncomfortable with how much of their vulnerability can show on their faces.

PERFORMANCE ANXIETY

Despite how comfortable they are in front of people, Yellows experience a lot of stress and anxiety if given too much planning time before they perform. They start doubting their abilities, asking nervous questions, sure that they are going to miss an important detail. Impromptu performances are much easier for them.

Yellows can carry a nervous, fluttery energy when they are unsure about something. This anxiety can come from small, everyday things or from larger dilemmas. They will gather information in order to feel informed and qualified for whatever they are dealing with. Unfortunately, they can assume the role of victim if they are not careful; assuming that everyone else has answers that they themselves cannot find. In these moments, it is helpful for Yellows to move their bodies, exercise, or do something else physically active. Answers and peace come to Yellows through movement.

PROLIFIC KINESTHETIC ARTISTS

Creation and art of all kinds are play for Yellows. Because they are kinesthetic and naturally optimistic, they are adventurous when creating art. They do not see why you would not create something out of 3D materials. Art is another form of play and they can become prolific visual artists. Yellows use their bodies to create so many things, like art, money, relationships, and adventures for the rest of us.

FANTASTIC SALESPEOPLE

Yellows can sell anything they can demonstrate. Sales can be a real draw for Yellows because it allows them to interact with people. They love helping people by showing them how to do things. They can sell ideas, products, and self-improvement aids, but are especially good at selling anything relating to the body—health food or products, exercise, sports, or any type of physical adventure. Also, in sales, they can do as much or as little as they want, which appeals to the loose schedule of Yellows.

Yellows initially take rejection personally, but eventually conquer that fear and replace it with a dogged determination. Yellows have unmatchable optimism. If they believe something can help others, then they do not care how many people reject it.

> *"Success is buried
> on the other side of rejection."*
> Anthony Robbins

If they believe in a person, then no one can change that. Yellows are amazingly loyal and committed friends and companions. When you are down there is no better gift than a Yellow friend. They never stop believing or encouraging their loved ones.

HOPEFUL LIGHTS
It gives Yellows immense satisfaction to bring joy to others. They have the gift of hope and they cannot help but spread it to others. Being bearers of hope is one of their true callings and purposes in life—whether they are conscious of it or not. They naturally lighten up heavy situations. Their light seems to make them incapable of despair and, gratefully, their light is contagious.

CHARISMATIC
Yellows are charismatic. Others are drawn to the heat and the joy that seems to resonate from every inch of their bodies. We all like to feel good in our bodies, but it is not natural for most of us to find consistent peace there. Yellows love their bodies and they teach the rest of us to enjoy our own bodies to the fullest extent.

ACCEPTING & OPEN
Yellows are accepting of themselves and others. They are also willing to try new things. Naturally open-minded

people, they are generally up for anything others want to do.

Because of their easy-going demeanor, they are able to motivate others to try many things they might otherwise avoid. They influence and challenge others through joy and fun. They are fantastic youth leaders, but can shift easily to interact with children or adults.

They are great in rehabilitation centers, working with troubled teens, teaching physical obstacle courses or leading any kind of high-adventure excursion. They can have many and varied types of careers if they can move about freely, create fun, talk, interact, and play with others. They are a welcome addition to any organization because they raise morale for the whole group.

THEIR GUT IS A SECOND BRAIN
Yellow bodies are like a highly active second brain. More specifically, their solar plexuses are networks of frantic activity, broadcasting information to them about themselves, others, and their environment, much of the time. Few others can relate to how much Yellows experience in their guts.

Yellows get mountains of information through their stomachs. They have all the gut reactions to the extreme. They just know an answer to something and say it is from their guts. They get butterflies, nausea, and too much movement in their stomachs when nervous or excited. Their stomachs get tied up in knots, and they say, "I can't eat because I'm too nervous." All of the sayings we use to describe an increase of stress in our bodies, positive or negative, primarily apply to Yellows.

Their bodies are constantly communicating to them, and sometimes it is hard for them to hear anything else.

HEIGHTENED SENSORY SYSTEM
They experience a lot of sensory data in their guts, but their entire bodies are often flooded with stimuli as well. One way they manage the input is by expending high energy in physical activities. There is an important input-output energy exchange that they have to work for in order to stay balanced. If they do not, Yellows can feel really agitated or depressed.

Yellows have bodies that react strongly to stimuli. If the average person has a moderately addictive response to chocolate, Yellows' responses will be extreme. Their chemical and physiological reactions are heightened. Addictions are created much more easily in their organism.

FRETTERS
For all of their tendencies to bring joy, Yellows are also worriers and fretters—not usually about deep things, but rather about immediate discomforts and disappointments.

When the rest of us begin to understand the high sensory communication going on in their bodies, it is a little easier to see why. They tend to verbally complain and become a bit self-centered and even whiney at these times. In all of their fretting what they are usually asking is for a confirmation that they are doing fine and that they are getting it right.

The truth of the matter is, Yellows just need things to be enjoyable and if they are too stressful, or too rigid, they feel a bit off-kilter and too much pressure.

ENCOURAGE & LOVE THEM

Sometimes it is difficult to take Yellows seriously, for all their play. That reaction is one of the few sources that cause Yellows deep emotional pain. Rejection is very difficult for Yellows in relationships, but also in other areas of their lives.

Some other personalities do not see the concrete value in the childlike demeanor of Yellows. The thing to remember, however, is that life without Yellows would be like an eternal dusk. They add immense warmth to the human experience, and heat is not just nice, it is essential to all life. It is also important to remember the perspective we gain when a little "light" is present.

To love Yellows, touch them, hug them, praise them and then, most importantly, play with them. To do this is to show them true appreciation for the light they so relentlessly share with us. Like puppies, little gestures of love and affection go a long way in gaining their loyalty and love.

If you have a Yellow in your life, don't take them for granted. Appreciate and praise them, and give gratitude for your good fortune that they are in your life. They are a gift, and we need to take care not to use them. We also need to acknowledge the balance they bring to our complicated, ego-driven, overly busy world.

If you find yourself flooded by their energy (that is always turned on, volume up) do not tell them to shut down but, rather, be responsible for your own boundaries. Create some temporary physical space between you. Give yourself adequate time alone. Then you will appreciate your interactive time with a Yellow so much more.

YELLOW FAMOUS PEOPLE*
Ronald Reagan—former U.S. president
John F. Kennedy (Blue-Amber)—former U.S. President
Steven R. Covey (Violet)—thought leader, speaker & author
Anthony Robbins (Violet)—thought leader, speaker & author
Will Smith—actor & musician
Lucille Ball—actor & comedian
Jim Carrey—actor & comedian
Sandra Bullock—actor
Conan O'Brien—talk show host & comedian
Angelina Jolie (Indigo)—actor
Travis Pastrana (Orange)—motorsports competitor & stuntman

Curious George

*Parentheses signify the secondary part of their main Aura Personality.

THE PHYSICAL-ENVIRONMENT FAMILY

~

AURA PERSONALITIES

The Physical Environment Aura Personalities

The Physical Environment Aura Personalities are the independent individualists. They walk their own walk, talk their own talk, and are completely unbound by tradition or social expectations.

The Physical Environment Aura Personalities are kinesthetic, but they are primarily spatial learners. Everything for them is about interacting with the three-dimensional planes of our world. They make manifest in the physical realm. They are production-based. They enjoy making things manifest, over conceptualizing things.

Physical Environment Aura Personalities experience life primarily through surveying, exploring and manipulating the terrain and raw materials of this planet, each in their own domain, focused on their particular interests. They are the Makers.

The Physical Environment Aura Personalities are:

REDS
ORANGES
MAGENTAS

~

THE RED
AURA PERSONALITY

The Landlord

"Lazily scratching his back on the rough bark of the old snag, he appeared unaware of the people frozen in their track so close by. But he had little to fear from any creature and was simply ignoring them. …The bear tired of his activity—or his itch was satisfied—and he stretched to his full height, walked on hind legs a few paces, then dropped on all four legs. …For all his great size, the cave bear was basically a peaceful creature and rarely attacked unless he was annoyed."
From *The Clan of the Cave Bear*, By Jean M. Auel

SURVEYORS

Reds are masters of the physical world. Hyper-aware of their surroundings, they maintain their bearings and have a clear picture of them at all times, including their own property and properties within their vicinity; in their home turf or wherever they may be visiting. Reds keep their eyes open for the rest of us.

Because they know their physical surroundings so well, they are the first to notice anything out-of-the-ordinary. Items out-of-place or missing. A stranger in the neighborhood or any other danger will quickly catch the attention of a Red. You can sleep better if you know you have a Red for a neighbor.

OWNERS OF THE EARTH

This vigilance is not born of fear but of dominion. Reds are the natural stewards of the land and they own the physical world. Not only do they survey all the land they see, they also work, till and transform it. They are not in the least intimidated by the earth. It is their playground and laboratory. They are amongst the stones, digging deep into the earth, or the waves, challenging the sea. They are builders, original trailblazers, and frontiersmen.

In a way the rest of us recognize Reds as our landlords—the true masters of the land. Reds were probably involved with the architecture of the world before and during its physical manifestation. We look to them to lead us on the physical plane, knowing they understand the earth better than anyone.

Reds do not even have to ask for respect from others- we give it immediately. We find Reds reassuring in their groundedness and naturally defer to their authority about the physical realm.

LABORERS
Over millennia, Reds have built society brick-by-brick, road-by-road, and railway-by-railway. They are the laborers—naturally strong, sturdy, stable and robust. They create the foundation on which we build our lives.

STRONG CONSTITUTIONS
Reds have strong physical constitutions. Their bodies can handle far more wear-and-tear than most people throughout their lives. They do not break easily. However, they do need to be somewhat mindful of their seeming infallibility because the day of reckoning comes for Reds who eat and do whatever they want with their bodies. It usually shows up in their backs and joints first, and then system conditions and disease show up later. But Reds are extremely thick-skinned and you will find them undertaking strenuous manual labor feats well into old age.

> *"I think retirement's for old people."*
> Harrison Ford

NEED TO FEEL USEFUL
Reds handle things in the physical realm with confidence and ease. They need to feel useful and are capable of any type of physical labor to demonstrate their usefulness. They know how to work.

RUGGED INDEPENDENT INDIVIDUALISTS
Nobody can work as hard as Reds; but they choose how and when they labor. They are very independent, rugged individualists. They are decisive and cannot be persuaded or coaxed away from what they decide for anything.

Reds are not going to do what they do not want to do-period. End of discussion (to write in their style of communication).

SIMPLE, STRONG, STRAIGHTFORWARD

Reds see themselves as they are—simple, strong, straightforward, and capable and doing their part. They do not try to fancy themselves up to be more than that. Reds feel absolutely no pressure to conform to anyone else's expectations.

> *"I'm not a facelift person.
> I am what I am."*
> Robert Redford

Much of the complexity of the world is seen for the nonsense that it is by Reds. They call it how they see it. If you want to be heard by Reds then give it to them straight and do not dress it up.

Reds are the no-nonsense Aura Personalities and tend to say things as they are, often to the chagrin of those around them. They are usually unaware of their lack of tact and if someone takes offense to this that is no reason for them to take back what they say.

There is a general feeling of "toughen up" and "suck it up" pressure when you are around Reds. The tenderhearted do not tend to keep close company with abrasive Reds. Harrison Ford exemplifies this in an interview with the British newspaper *The Telegraph* when asked if he is grumpy: *"Am I grumpy?" Harrison Ford ponders the idea, and acknowledges: "I might be." Then the gruff and occasionally acerbic actor adds: "But I think maybe sometimes it's misinterpreted. I've always been an independent... So, if I'm grumpy, then call me grumpy. I'm all right with that."*

CONCRETE THINKERS
Reds would rather talk about concrete things over principles or ideas. In general they are uncomfortable and even bored with conversation that gets analytical or too abstract. They keep things real and conversation light. To accomplish this they can often be self-deprecating and teasing of others. They have a good sense of humor and will use it to lighten things up.

LONG-WINDED, FACT-BASED TALKERS
Reds enjoy hearing and telling stories and can be quite long-winded in recounting details of physical descriptions and factual events. Their comfortableness in that drawn-out, timeless space, telling us how their cattle are faring, or retelling each detail of their child's baseball game, is something we savor about reds. They run on their own time clock and do not feel that they owe anyone an explanation for the way they operate. We like and admire them for their innate self-respect.

FEARLESS
Even during calamity or crisis, Reds keep the hysteria down. They don't get caught up in the fear, nor do they buy into our modern anxiety. They are too grounded for that. They are part of the rugged land and take all things in stride. They are nonplussed by the hustle, bustle and unnatural stopwatch pacing of our modern world. And, although they are not much esteemed in our modern culture for their contributions, we would float away without their solid constancy.

ROOTED TO THE EARTH
Reds are like mountains and forests, enduring and existing outside of social constructs. They continually draw us back to the land, back to the more natural,

grounded pace they innately obey. As the manmade, so-called "tornados" of modern life whirl about, sucking us into stress, anxiety and dis-ease, Reds are fixed in place. They are rooted within themselves like giant sequoias, sending roots deep into the earth. Reds hold firmly to the ground and maintain their footing like Stonehenge or the Pyramids in Egypt.

GUARDIANS & PROTECTORS
Reds are like the land, obedient children of Father Time. Slowly carved and altered over eons of time, like the Grand Canyon or the Amazon River basin. Reds are undaunted by disaster and can assist the masses during crises because of their grounded natures. Everyone feels less worried and safer around Reds. They allow the rest of us to let our guard down a bit because they never do. They are the guardians, the pillars of strength in unnatural, unsteady times where most of us live disobedient to nature's rhythm and pacing.

BRAVE BUT IMPETUOUS
Reds are fearless. They are willing to confront just about anyone or anything that appears menacing or threatening to them or anyone else. They are courageous, probably to a fault, and tend to jump-the-gun into action before they are clear of all the facts. Because of their innate bravery, Reds may find themselves in unsavory settings or confronting unsavory people but, because of their thick skin, they do not erode easily and bounce back even after tremendous trial.

The Red politician, John McCain, is an amazing example of this kind of bravery when, after five-and-a-half years as a prisoner of war, two of which were in solitary confinement, he surfaced not in defeat but in victory.

McCain went on to serve his country for several decades, first as a Navy captain and then as a United States Senator.

PUPPIES & BEARS
In general, Reds have the playful physical energy and intentions of puppies coupled with the strength, weight and effect of bears, and they are generally oblivious to that fact. Like bears, Reds can bellow. And, like bears, they can blow through things causing destruction in their wake, hurting things and people just by the sheer force of their presence. Like a bumbling bear, they cause landslides that wipe out whole trees in their path, causing all other animals to run and hide in an effort to avoid getting caught underfoot.

Despite their strong presence, Reds wouldn't harm a flea without pretense. Reds are often the greatest protectors of children, underdogs and defenseless people. They can automatically assume immediate and constant protection from Reds. They are the guardians and protectors. And the gifts required to fulfill that calling make them rough and even offensive at times to the rest of us.

It is important to understand why Reds are as harsh as they are. And, although they can learn to soften, their rough and sturdy exterior was no mistake in design and serves all of us in essential ways.

UNCOMFORTABLE WITH EMOTION
Reds are very comfortable and natural in their role as protector, but they are not comfortable with many other social roles. They keep an emotional distance from others, in general, because they are wary of emotions—their own and others. Emotions are unfamiliar and

intangible, so they keep their own close. Very few people, if any, are allowed into their inner world, and they do not ever spend much time there.

> *"They say marriages are made in heaven.
> But so is thunder and lightning."*
> Clint Eastwood

In many ways, Reds are like very big two-year-olds when it comes to emotional expression. They lash out when hurt. They are extremely uncomfortable with strong emotions and might run and hide when they surface. Like two-year-olds, Reds often use physical means to express strong emotions, including closeness, love, fear, anger and sorrow. They do this because they are unsure how to manifest emotions in any other way.

An older woman described a childhood interaction with her Red husband: when they were young children, walking home from grammar school one day, he playfully tackled her to the ground like a bear cub. He thought he was being affectionate, but she was shocked and dismayed. The gesture was almost lost on her. But, years later, when he more appropriately courted and married her, she recalls this story with affection and admits that he still struggles to express strong emotion in any other way but physically.

BOSSY, COARSE & LOUD AT TIMES
When Reds get angry they can be very coarse and loud. Like growling bears, they can be terrifying to children and others. Others end up feeling like punished two-year-olds in the presence of Red anger. Luckily, that anger is infrequent. It actually takes quite a lot of ammunition for Reds to build up to angry outbursts. People often think they are mad or irritated by their

tone, because the way they speak is abrupt and rough. Unless they know them well, others can never quite tell if Reds are angry or not.

Reds tend to be bossy and give orders. They do not feel obligated to explain or justify their expectations to others. They easily notice what others should be doing and tell them to do it. They even expect the strong independence and self-sufficiency so natural in them from everyone else.

TOUGH LOVE & STRONG WORK ETHIC
Although infants do not hold much interest for Reds, they find great satisfaction watching as children mature and become more and more physically capable. They enjoy teaching children that labor is play, and that building dexterity and strength is fun. Reds have the ability to teach all of life's lessons through such means.

In parenting and mentoring they do much better with teenagers than young children. Teenagers are open to learning from strong independent Reds as they work to unveil their own independence. Reds feel like sturdy oaks and an anchor in an otherwise unstable world. Even if Red love is tough love, teenagers respect this, knowing what they see is what they will always get because Reds are so consistent with who they are.

The real difficulty Reds encounter in mentoring young people is in the emotional realm. Because of their insensitivity to the inner world of others, Reds can sometimes feel very out-of-touch, or communicate through their behavior that there is no place for emotion. Teenagers will seek out others to learn those kinds of lessons.

ACTION-ORIENTED DO-ERS

People immediately respect Reds because Reds get things done without having to talk or overthink. In fact, Reds feel very impatient with talk and instead, move immediately to action.

To Reds, talk is cheap; action is everything. This is a good motto for many situations, but sometimes considerations are required but, instead, Reds act brashly before they have heard all of the details.

> *"Sometimes if you want to see a change for the better, you have to take things into your own hands."*
> Clint Eastwood

Red men are the iconoclastic males cast as leading men in films for most of the twentieth century. Many men think they are supposed to be like Red men because of such role models. Demonstrating the idea that tough, strong, and independent are the male ideal, even if their own gifts and proclivities lie in other arenas.

Red women, on the other hand, can really struggle to fit in because they are so physically strong, and often uninterested in many typically female roles. They find great satisfaction in mechanics, construction and farming, as well as other labor-intensive roles.

Red women can certainly run a household, but it will be in a practical, no-nonsense fashion. Reds do not apologize for themselves. They come to acceptance about any role they are in, but can feel a bit set apart from other women and society in general because of their non-traditional demeanors.

PRIDEFUL & RESISTANT TO CHANGE
Reds do not feel guilty often. Reds feel justified. They are right and, even if they are not, who cares (as they would say), since they only answer to themselves. Reds do not feel that they owe explanations to anyone and, actually, they do not feel that they "owe" anyone anything. Reds can be above the law in their own minds, if they are not careful, and this can get them into trouble.

Strong and immovable as oaks, they can be equally prideful and resistant to change. But with the wisdom of all great trees, they have the sense to carve out their own lives with as much independence and room as they might need.

PRACTICAL INTELLIGENCE
Reds intelligence is pure unadulterated common sense. They always default to the thing that is the most obvious. Reds understand practicality. They see through frivolous detail to what is and are then able to rapidly summarize the situation. Occasionally subtler details are missed, but this decreases over time.

LIVE & LET LIVE
With *live and let live* as their general motto for life, we all learn great lessons in self-sufficiency and self-respect dwelling amongst sturdy, grounded Reds.

RED FAMOUS PEOPLE*
Cary Grant (Lavender)—actor
Gordon B. Hinckley (Violet)—Prophet
Robert Redford (Green)—actor & director
Hilary Swank—actor

Red ♦ THE LANDLORD

Harrison Ford—actor, volunteer search & rescue pilot
John McCain—U.S. Navy officer & politician
Gordon Ramsey—chef & restaurateur
Clint Eastwood—actor

Grizzly Adams
Johnny Appleseed
Tom Bombadil-from J.R.R. Tolkien's *Lord of the Rings*

*Parentheses signify the secondary part of their main Aura Personality.

~

THE ORANGE AURA PERSONALITY

The Summiteer

"An optimist is someone who goes after Moby Dick in a rowboat and takes the tartar sauce with him."
Zig Ziglar

NO-LIMIT SUMMITEERS
Picture a world without Olympians, explorers or summiteers, without the people that push beyond the boundaries of what we previously believed to be the limit of physical capability. That would be our world without Oranges.

Although it seems there are fewer Oranges in the world, this is only because they are not sitting around social circles discussing philosophy, politics, labor, or personality types. In fact, Oranges are not sitting around anywhere unless, of course, it is their campfire at the base of Mount Everest just before their final ascent, or in a trailer resting after a kamikaze stunt.

PLAYGROUND IS EARTH, SKY & WATER

Oranges live to challenge and be challenged by the physical planes of earth, sky, and water. Nature is where they generally reside, but not in peaceful bliss. Oranges appreciate nature's majesty, but they are far more focused on conquering and defying it through their physical prowess than enjoying its beauty.

> *"A ship is safe in harbor,*
> *but that's not what ships are for."*
> William G.T. Shedd

DAREDEVILS & RISK-TAKERS

There is no such thing as fear for Oranges. Adrenaline, yes; fear, no. Oranges are internally driven to find physical challenge. Stunt people, big wave surfers, mountain climbers, skydivers, and base jumpers usually have Orange in their auric field, even if it is not their first aura personality. If they do have it, the call to risk-taking is loud and will not be ignored. Oranges are not happy if they are not taking risks or challenging their previous records of personal excellence.

Risk seeking can easily turn into addiction for Oranges. They are addicted to the challenge and the attending adrenaline. Oranges take any challenge and go bigger, faster, stronger, deeper, or higher. They turn everything up a notch. They have to watch this need for increased risk because everything else can fall to the wayside if they are not careful, including their safety.

AURA PERSONALITIES

"Freedom lies in being bold."
Robert Frost

OLYMPIANS

Fortunately for Oranges, there are abundant outlets for them to explore their drive to physically overcome. Programs like the Olympic games, extreme sporting competitions, and even military roles, provide ample opportunity for them to self-actualize while simultaneously becoming an integral part of society. They can get paid for what they love to do and be part of organizations that value them for their single-minded focus and efforts.

All modern extreme sports have Orange personalities somewhere in their pioneering efforts, pushing them to great heights that the rest of us will then spend lifetimes trying to reach. Oranges are the gold standard in performance.

ROLE MODELS & PUBLIC FIGURES

Growing up, Oranges are generally misunderstood. Others expect them to be interested in traditional activities and do not understand their hyper-focus in one area of life. As Oranges age, others begin congratulating them for their persistence in their grandiose pursuits. Eventually, Oranges find great acceptance and encouragement for what they do, instead of feeling like a disappointment because of their single-minded ambitions.

We laud their feats as the standard to aspire to. We look up to Oranges, and even idolize them for their bravery and determination. We turn them into spokespeople, and public figures. We pay them to be role models and lifestyle endorsers for our own purposes. Oranges are fine in these roles and often take them on just so they can get more gear, tools, and training options for their particular pursuits.

Oranges are not afraid of the public, public attention, or fame. They can take notoriety in stride and use it for their benefit and as a way to shine in what they are.

PHYSICAL SELF-DISCIPLINE
Oranges need a high-risk, physical challenge all of the time, or at least need to be planning and preparing for one in the near future. They are admirable in their meticulous discipline in preparing for events. No one can focus and eliminate all other distractions like Oranges can.

> *"Spectacular achievements are always preceded by unspectacular preparation."*
> Roger Staubach

Oranges will train and work to achieve their particular objectives. Everything else in life becomes secondary to their physical preparations or personal pursuits.

SINGLE-MINDED & DRIVEN
Others greatly admire the single-mindedness of Oranges. The passion and focus they operate from are breathtaking and quite attractive. Oranges, like their Aura Personality hue, are like wildfire. There is no stopping their flame and drive to exceed previous records.

> *"Courage and perseverance have a magical talisman, before which difficulties disappear and obstacles vanish into air."*
> John Quincy Adams

Oranges are the kind of people who go to the moon without glancing back, or train to hold their breath underwater longer than anyone had before them. They push and strive toward personal physical excellence almost without awareness of anything else going on in the world. The world goes through its trials, tying itself up in conflicts and strife, but Oranges stand apart from all of that. They inhabit a different world, one without politics, conflict or trial.

OWN THE EARTH, SEA & SKY

Oranges have a unique bird's-eye view of societies and cultures. They see the planet as a whole, for what it actually is, instead of as a place with separate political entities jostling for power and dominion. Oranges know the planet is really their own. They are the ones really taking advantage of all it has to offer by way of land, sky and bodies of water. The entire world is literally an enormous playground for them.

Oranges feel that the earth and its resources are here for them. They do not feel guilty for dirt biking through pristine forests, or placing metal climbing spikes along walls of rock. Oranges are using the earth. They are taking full advantage of all the earth has to offer and they do not really understand why the rest of us would spend so much time, energy, or resources constructing buildings and social structures when we could just acquire all the learning we need from nature, by using the elements and our bodies.

DISREGARD FOR AUTHORITY & TRADITION

Being so detached from normal societal aims, Oranges have a natural disregard for authority and tradition. Authority figures can be seen as one more force of nature to be subdued or challenged. This is really just pent up energy to be explored and relieved by getting into nature and achieving their personal physical goals of stamina, strength, and drive.

Along with authority, traditions do not really apply to Oranges either. They are too focused on their own objectives to be concerned with tradition or societal norms. This can be frustrating for their families and friends. Although they admire their Orange loved ones, they are saddened to feel emotionally distant from them.

RELATIONSHIPS CAN BE SECONDARY
Just like Reds, emotions and emotional closeness are unfamiliar to Oranges because they are intangible and seemingly undefined. Oranges desire close relationships at times, but the call to physical challenge is often much louder than the soft voice of close relationships.

If their partner can understand the drive of Oranges, then the relationship can succeed. You just might find that they have partially chosen you because of how you help them in their personal goals of physical challenge. Relationships often become secondary to them. You would have to recognize that fact and come to terms with it in order to find happiness in your relationship with them. Otherwise, you will just be in their way, so it will not be able to last long.

Oranges are marching to a beat separate and apart from the drumroll the rest of us follow. They can be seen as self-centered and distant because of their single-mindedness. Their souls simply need challenge- extreme challenge. They are compelled to seek it. Oranges have to find something in the physical world to defy, or they feel lost.

FLYING SOLO
Oranges fly solo. They are often involved in activities and adventures that they experience alone. They choose activities, sports, careers and lifestyles where they will have all the room they need to accomplish their personal objectives. They do not seem to need very much by way of companionship or friendship, and they can be without companionship for much longer periods of time than most of us.

Their most common relationships are partners in crime, people with the same passions and drive for personal achievement. Green-Ambers, Yellows and Reds often join Oranges on the frontlines of risk-taking and challenge. Oranges develop camaraderie and feel understood by these people far more than by anyone else. Of course Oranges take it a step further than their peers, and all are aware how much greater their commitment is to achieve their goals. Most other personalities are unwilling to sacrifice all other things in the name of such pursuits.

The rest of society and its customs are strange and foreign to Oranges. They see how they are apart and separate. They do not worry about this fact, but they do notice it.

TAKE US TO NEW HEIGHTS & FRONTIERS
Many of us cannot relate to this instinctive drive Oranges have to defy what, to the rest of us, seem to be the natural limits of the body. Oranges are here to break records as well as the boundaries of what we previously

believed about our physical capabilities. But there is something extremely valuable to the collective psyche in knowing the boundaries we once thought unbreakable can be overcome.

Oranges conquer those pre-existing limits. They show us what is possible. They are the beings that represent, on the physical plane, that everything is possible.

> *"Life is not about discovering our talents;*
> *it is about pushing our talents to the limit*
> *and discovering our genius."*
> Robert Brault

ORANGE FAMOUS PEOPLE*
Jill Stevens-Shepherd (Green-Amber)—National Guard Medic, former Miss Utah, marathon runner
Ernest Shakleton (Green-Amber)—Irish polar explorer
Edmund Hillary—mountaineer, explorer, philanthropist
Evel Knievel (Green)—American daredevil, entertainer

Many Olympians
Explorers
Military people (especially in high-risk divisions)
Extreme sport athletes
Big wave surfers
Summiteers
Rock and ice climbers
Base-jumpers

*Parentheses signify the secondary part of their main Aura Personality.

THE MAGENTA
AURA PERSONALITY

The Creator

"When I am traveling in a carriage, or walking after a good meal, or during the night when I cannot sleep; it is on such occasions that ideas flow best and most abundantly... Nor do I hear in my imagination the parts successively; I hear them all at once. What a delight this is! All this inventing, this producing, takes place in a pleasing, lively dream."
Wolfgang Amadeus Mozart

PROLIFIC CREATORS
Magentas are the physical conduits for creation. They are in a state of putting their imaginations into the physical realm nearly all the time. Creations burst forth from

them. Magentas are the people who can recreate a thunder and lightning storm and transform it into a magnificent symphony in a single sitting.

> *"Everything you can imagine is real."*
> Pablo Picasso

There really are no limits on what can be created by Magentas. They can be a painter, and then pick up and learn the guitar in a night. They can be an architect, and then make a beautiful sculpture on their first try. Magentas are extremely capable, gifted people.

Their capability, and their willingness to share their imaginations, is what they offer the world. Magentas teach us to connect to our own imaginations and give them more value and heed.

> *"One of the most important gifts*
> *we have is imagination.*
> *It makes up 95 per cent of our minds,*
> *it's our greatest asset, our best friend,*
> *and, in some cases, if we're not careful,*
> *our worst enemy."*
> Johnny Depp

Prolific is a serious understatement to describe the creative manifestations of Magentas. They run at a pace of creation as if the world is going to end before they can get the multitudes of their creations out. The creative energy pulsing through them is so charged, there is nothing for them to do but manifest.

> *"Only put off until tomorrow*
> *what you are willing to die*
> *having left undone."*
> Pablo Picasso

Magentas are unaware of how astounded the rest of us are by their high volume of creative output. They are not able to be objective about themselves in this way. If you do not offer input, they will ask for verbal affirmations and confirmations about their creations. They want to know that what they are doing is worthwhile. As prolific as they are, Magentas still need a lot of assurances from others.

Magentas can use their creativity in a variety of settings, but you will find them most frequently in artistic pursuits like composing and performing music, acting, doing physical comedy, painting, sculpting, designing, drafting, or creating large-scale land art.

STRONG CONSTITUTIONS & STAMINA
Magentas have strong physical constitutions and stamina matched only by other Physical Environment Aura Personalities. They use their physical strength to construct, build, create and spread their creations to the masses. They are tireless. It is as if their minds are in a creation state that will not release them until they have manifested their ideas into physical reality.

EXPRESSIVE & INTERACTIVE
When Magentas are not creating; they are using their bodies and words for animated expression and interaction. Magentas demand attention. They do not know how to be wallflowers. They flit about the room, stirring up energy wherever they go, and everyone is aware of them.

Magentas are sassy, spunky, and shoot electricity into the room from their centers and out through their fingers and toes. They are fun and physically interactive and often touch others when they speak to them.

FULLY ENGAGED & FULLY DISENGAGED

Magentas are interesting companions because they so fully engage you one minute, getting right in your space and demanding complete attention. Then, in the next moment, they are off, having moved on to something or someone else.

At other times, rather than abruptly switching the object of their engagement, they will completely disengage. They are right with you, present, paying attention, closely engaged, and then, suddenly, they are not. This usually happens during their times of creation. If Magentas are working on something, they physically flit around, as always, but it is as if you are no longer in the room. "What? Did you say something?" they'll ask, suddenly realizing they are not alone.

INTIMACY CAN BE TRICKY

Needless to say, Magentas do not attract many intimate relationships at a time because others have to be willing to shift with their erratic behavior. Magentas simultaneously want closeness as well as freedom. They are similar to Lavenders in this way, but Magentas are much more engaged when they are with someone than Lavenders are. This fully engaged or completely separate dynamic is intense and makes Magentas a hard read for a lot of people. Although it is possible, others find it difficult to see how they fit into the intricate, constantly moving and changing lives of Magentas.

Most of us wonder how there is any order or structure in the lives of Magentas. Magentas are on the extreme end of nontraditional. Societal norms do not dictate their actions in any way.

LOYAL, ACCEPTING & NONJUDGMENTAL

With relationships, it is a question of whether or not others can accept the nontraditional parameters of Magentas. Interestingly, Magentas feel no need to push what they are onto anyone else. They do not need others to be any other way than exactly how they are, and would appreciate this treatment in return. Those who can accept the unconventional lifestyle and thoughts of Magentas can have exceptional relationships with them.

Magentas are loyal to their loved ones. When you are in a relationship with them, you feel their loyalty to you and dependency on your love.

Magentas could have close relationships with many people. They love the feeling of supportive people in their lives, as well as giving their love and support to others. They feel sad that others let their differences get in the way of loving relationships.

MELODRAMATIC & TRANSPARENT

Magentas are very melodramatic. They show their moods clearly and vacillate between happy, carefree, and exuberant, to openly moping, downtrodden, and depressed. Their moods show in their whole bodies. Unhappy: slumping, hanging head, slack arms; Upset: folded arms, puffed up chest, pursed lips; Happy: outstretched arms, running around, smiles and words of joy flying freely from their lips.

*"Comedy is
acting out optimism."*
Robin Williams

Magentas appreciate the shocking and unexpected, and have playful, odd, quirky senses of humor. Not everyone gets the humor of Magentas, but that does not stop them from putting it out there.

TALKATIVE & EXPRESSIVE
Magentas use their whole bodies to communicate all that is going on for them internally. They are great models for animation, as well as amazing physical comedians and actors, because they are so exaggerated and emotionally expressive in their body language and facial expressions.

Maybe Magentas are showing us the true way, the more honest way of living in a body filled with emotions. Maybe we would internalize less stress if we let our bodies demonstrate our moods as actively and fully as Magentas express.

Magentas are naturally talkers and are very verbal about their musings, thoughts and opinions. They are bright, descriptive and energetic. They use strong statements and wide gestures to describe their opinions and feelings: I hate, I detest, I deplore, I adore, I'm absolutely in love with, et cetera. There is no middle ground for Magentas in terms of expression. They express fully.

BODY CONFIDENT
Magentas are beyond body confident, because they are too busy gesturing and expressing to even think about what they look like. Others find this very endearing and attractive about them. We watch them and wonder how they can be so free, unaffected, spontaneous, and playful in their movement.

AVANT-GARDE

Magentas like shocking things, the avant-garde, and they like to surround themselves with people and environments that stimulate their creativity and provide their imaginations with fuel.

Magentas adore people. They feel a little shy about who they are around others, but they love people too much to stay away for long. Magentas like to learn and they learn much by observing and interacting with others.

ECLECTIC, SELF-TAUGHT LEARNERS

Magentas are bright, kinesthetic learners, but utilize other faculties to learn as well. They are able to gather seemingly random information to create their own ideal, eclectic, tailor-made, learning environments. They are also able to get what they need from formal education, if they are allowed to. Even though the arts and creativity are electives in most school systems, Magentas will hone in and get all that they need from those existing programs.

STRONG WORK ETHIC

Magentas know how to work. Their work ethic around their interests and creations is significant. What they spend their time on is not always viewed as worthwhile, however. It is much easier to say that Gaudi or Picasso or Mozart used their time well and were prolific, productive artists because their work has transcended their deaths. We can see the fruits of their labors. But, it is much more difficult to call the work of Magentas useful until it is making money for them or gets noticed on a wider scale.

Magenta ♦ THE CREATOR

> *"Inspiration exists,
> but it has to find us working."*
> Pablo Picasso

Magentas are busy doing what they do, busier than most people, but they need to be careful not to judge the value of their work based on society's response to it. With time, society always responds to the creative output of Magentas. It has to because there is usually so much of it.

Magentas are some of the few types of artists that will make significant sums of money for their creativity all throughout their lives. But there is a period of waiting for a response from the world for all of their creative efforts. That can be a difficult period for Magentas and they need to not give up hope.

MAGENTA FAMOUS PEOPLE*
Wolfgang Amadeus Mozart—composer
Antonio Gaudi—Spanish artist
Pablo Picasso—Spanish artist
William Shakespeare (Red-Amber)—poet, actor & dramatist
Steve Jobs—entrepreneur, designer & inventor
Diane Keaton—actor
Robin Williams—actor & comedian
Johnny Depp—actor
Tim Burton—artist & filmmaker

*Parentheses signify the secondary part of their main Aura Personality.

AURA PERSONALITIES

THE MENTAL FAMILY
~

AURA PERSONALITIES

The Mental Aura Personalities

The Mental Aura Personalities take in life experiences and learning first through their minds. They have to first make logical sense of any situation, even traumatic ones, before they can respond. They bring level-headedness and reason to every situation. Most things can be deduced to business for them. They are natural administrators, creating structure and order for us all. They find the rational way to solve any problem.

The Mental Aura Personalities are trying to get their "mental" bearings all of the time. They are constantly scanning for cues and clues. They learn rapidly, in an orderly fashion and are able to teach what they learn.

The Mental Aura Personalities are mental architects. They are constructing society through sound logic and planning. And then they are willing to hold up the support beams of that society indefinitely.

The Mental Aura Personalities are:

AMBERS
GREENS

~

THE AMBER AURA PERSONALITY

The Judge

> *"...The real world can only be apprehended intellectually...knowledge cannot be transferred from teacher to student, but rather that education consists in directing student's minds toward what is real and important and allowing them to apprehend it for themselves..."*
>
> From *Allegory of The Cave*,
> Book *VII The Republic*, By Plato

ACTIVE QUESTIONERS & LEARNERS
There are no more tenacious learners than Ambers. Operating in a state of perpetual, active learning, Ambers ask questions and acquire information everywhere they

go. Different from distracted and distant mental Greens, Ambers are present and engaged in conversations of procedures, ideas, debate, facts, events, or even just verbal banter. They talk through as they go, sharing what they know with others. You might find them talking through the actions of a child or a stranger you are observing together. They are interested in anything, if not to incorporate it into their lives, then just to make sense of it.

Ambers are not always talking, however. They are often observing. Making sense. Accumulating data. Making calculations. They wait and watch and wonder, periodically asking questions. They are comfortable with the mundane because everything is information that grows their knowledge bank. They are in a state of mental tracking most of the time.

WORDS ARE THEIR PLAYGROUND
Ambers love riddles, associations, plays-on-words, and puzzles. Debate is fun and logic games are leisure for them.

Ambers are engaged and somewhat emotionally charged during discussions. To some of us they appear argumentative or even negative, but to them they are just discussing a topic, fleshing out an issue, or simply having fun watching how words can affect others. They can stay fairly neutral when they debate. What feels like conflict to some, is actually a stimulating tension that Ambers enjoy.

Ambers can be wry and acerbic, with dry senses of humor that are saturated with sarcasm. They cannot resist verbal banter. They can dish it, and can take it, as the saying goes, since they are not overly sensitive. And, although they are interested in obtaining information, they are not particularly gossipy or fickle in conversation. Gaining information is not just for curiosity's sake. Ambers love information for its potential usefulness, and conversation with others is one of their quickest ways to gain that information.

People that actually enjoy the sample test questions in preparation for the LSAT (Law School Assessment Test) are often Ambers. Words are their weapons, and they always fire them through logic and as much evidence as they can gather. Ambers can argue their way out of or into anything they set their minds to. It takes a lot to verbally intimidate them.

PRAGMATIC
If something is not useful, Ambers have a hard time seeing the point of it. Ambers are practical and information needs to have an application. This attitude bleeds into their material lives. They are frugal in that what they buy has to be justified. They can be penny-pinchers and even stingy if they are not mindful of this over-practicality.

> *"I have a great respect for money.*
> *I know how hard it is to earn and keep,*
> *especially with our diabolical taxes in Britain.*
> *I never get over the fact that sometimes I see more money*
> *being paid for a meal than my father earned in a week."*
> Sean Connery

Frugality serves Ambers in many ways except where loved ones are concerned because the needs of people often fall outside the lines of what is practical or frugal.

Matters of the heart do not always follow laws of accounting or a budget.

CREATORS OF MODERN EDUCATION
The Socratic and scientific methods, critical questioning, thinking, reasoning, and memorization are all offspring of Amber minds. These areas also form the foundation of our modern education system, which was created by them and, incidentally, for them. So, of course, Ambers are the most comfortable students and teachers within this current system, and Countless educators, and not a few college professors, have Amber Aura Personalities.

We are all familiar with Amber ways because their ways are clear, knowable, and logically expressed. Most of us have held them up as standards of excellence in education, at one time or another, as they so often set the achievement curve for high grades and high-test scores. Ambers test well because (a) they wrote the textbooks from which we are tested, the structure of what is on tests, and how tests are administered; and, (b) they are committed to paying the price of study, keeping up on homework, and staying on task.

Ambers experience intense satisfaction in accomplishing goals and the school system provides ample opportunities for them to achieve. They walk a fine line between achieving for personal excellence and external accolades. Pride is a temptation that is not easily overcome by Ambers since our society readily rewards so much of what they naturally accomplish.

RECORD KEEPERS
With minds that are precision instruments, Ambers gather, track and accumulate all kinds of data, even the

most mundane. They have incredible memories and serve as oral and written record keepers for the rest of us. They enjoy writing things down and want details in every step or part of a thing or idea in which they are involved, willing to record happenings to the minute.

SKEPTICAL DELIBERATORS

Ambers are infinitely patient, and willing to remain inconclusive much longer than the rest of us as they wait for facts, because nothing else will do in formulating conclusions. They deliberate and consider multiple sides of most issues.

Ambers are the natural skeptics and cynics, wary and untrusting of decisions reached too easily or quickly by others. So they wait and deliberate until they have finally been given enough information. Once they have it, Ambers are incredibly decisive, and it is very difficult to steer them away from their conclusions.

Ambers can be prideful in their perceptions and beliefs in this way, believing that the way they think is the only logical or "right" way since they go to much greater lengths to formulate those beliefs. They set themselves apart, and even above others in these ways. They have to watch their Egos probably more than any other personality. Their need to constantly learn more information is the one thing that keeps this tendency in check.

MEDIATORS & JUDGES

Ambers love all the facts to be laid out on the table. They wait patiently to acquire all the details they need. They remain removed and objective when gathering information.

Amber ♦ THE JUDGE

Ambers are not intimidated by much, and can even bite back, if the situation so requires. Ambers can tolerate a lot of harsh and hostile input that would be taxing on many of the rest of us day-in-and day-out. But Ambers are thick-skinned. Things do not seem to penetrate into the realm of their feelings very easily. And they can definitely hold their own verbally. Ambers can, in fact, cut people off, cut-to-the-chase, and move-on, all in one breath. In some situations these are rough traits to be smoothed out and remedied. In others, they are the best, most essential traits to get a job done, ones that mediators and judges who are truly just would need to possess.

Both roles of mediator and judge often fall to Ambers. There are few others patient enough, emotionally removed enough, or composed enough to carry out the duties those roles require. Many of these professional skills can seem harsh or overly analytical in some settings, but are essential in others. Ambers hold the kind of objectivity societies need to maintain justice and order.

Ambers have to take care not to let their analytical tendencies, in words and demeanor, spill into their personal relationships. One of their lessons is learning how to have their words fit individual settings and particular people. Ambers enjoy this. It is one of their lifelong lessons.

SEEKERS OF ENLIGHTENMENT
Ambers are the truly critical thinkers challenging society with their questions, ever pushing the envelope to reach that edge of thought where illumination bursts through. Ambers live for those hard-earned moments of

intellectual clarity. For them, intellectual enlightenment is the highest aim.

> *"Men are more readily contented
> with no intellectual light than with a little;
> and wherever they have been taught
> to acquire some knowledge in order to please others,
> they have most generally gone on
> to acquire more, to please themselves."*
> From *Lacon*, Charles Caleb Colton

Ambers are not content to just sit and think about their enlightenment, they must act, and they tend to be on the extreme end of action. As doers, they are chomping at the bit, ever anticipating what they will accomplish next on their list of goals.

APPLY WHAT THEY LEARN

What Ambers learn, they apply. So when they find out that walking reduces heart disease, they schedule time and start walking, regularly. If they find out that going on a date with their spouse once a week helps marriages, that date will happen every week forever more.

> *"Knowing is not enough; we must apply.
> Willing is not enough; we must do."*
> Johann Wolfgang Goethe

STRIVING & DOING

Ambers strive for excellence, using the breadth of their acquired knowledge as a standard, and then they do what is expected. They, in turn expect the same of others, especially those within their realm of stewardship. Ambers need to take care in their expectations of others and note that all people have different contributions. We are not all striving toward the same end. What Ambers hold as the standard is not really what everyone else should be striving toward.

OBJECTIVE OBSERVER
Although it is difficult for Ambers to recognize that their standards are not everyone's; once they do, they can really help others achieve their particular goals. Ambers can always muster an objective perspective to any situation, once they get over the fact that their way is not the only way, that is.

Ambers are able to get over themselves once they put their minds to it. It is one of their greatest offerings to the rest of us. It is why we often hire them for their expertise, to guide us through our finances, our legal disputes, and to run our companies and other organizations. If they get a clear picture of what our contribution is—albeit different from their own—they make for amazing partners and team players.

INFLUENCE ALL SOCIAL CONSTRUCTS
From being able to check items off their to-do lists down to adding educational diplomas and awards to their walls of accomplishments, Ambers find great satisfaction in seeing things through for themselves and for others. They are accomplished individuals that infiltrate, influence and dominate our modern educational, business, political, and religious systems. We want them in those places because they are the most willing to tend the shop and manage the day-to-day affairs of life.

ACTIVE
Ambers are meticulous and fastidious in the way they live and set their priorities. Task-oriented and goal-

oriented, they keep the rest of us on target. They are tireless in their activity, endlessly going and doing. This is an interesting parallel lifestyle for people who are also so busy in their thoughts. It is as if high physical activity is fuel for the high mental activity of Ambers, and they love to see the results of that expended energy on both counts.

PLANNERS, NEED-TO-KNOW

From very young ages, Ambers keep their parents on their toes with their need for planned, regular activities and a constant need to know what is coming next. They can be incessant in asking for more and clearer details about the future.

Not knowing what to expect, or what is expected of them, is the single greatest source of stress and anxiety for Ambers, and they expend enormous amounts of energy to avoid being taken by surprise. Ambers become experts at this but, alas, their system is not fail-proof as the unexpected knocks suddenly and unawares even on their doors.

ADMINISTRATORS

Ambers are born creatures of habit, routine, schedules and day-planners. They are the best people to run any kind of organization, from a household to a corporation to a large government agency. Ambers are paying attention, tracking details and people, daily, systematically. They enjoy this kind of accounting.

Ambers need to constantly assess their bearings. They are like compasses constantly ascertaining north and comparing everything else to it. If they are clear on an organizations goals and objectives, they are able to consistently and steadily steer the whole ship towards true north.

> *"I am personally convinced that one person can be a change catalyst, a 'transformer' in any situation, any organization. Such an individual is yeast that can leaven an entire loaf. It requires vision, initiative, patience, respect, persistence, courage, and faith to be a transforming leader."*
> Stephen R. Covey

They naturally have gifts in administration. To borrow a religious analogy, Ambers are the active stewards of the vineyard, involved in the daily work, overseeing the labors of others, and giving an accounting to the master of the vineyard.

WHAT YOU SEE IS WHAT YOU GET
Ambers are fairly transparent. We can take them at their word. They are happier with an agenda, a to-do list, and if those around them can accept this then they are easy people to be around. You always know where they stand because they communicate it through the routines of their lives.

Ambers can be people who hang out in the background. This is not because they are shy or timid; they are just not center-of-attention people. When Ambers are ready to speak, however, they will speak.

Even though they do not need to voice all of their ideas, when Ambers are ready to speak they expect people to listen attentively and not interrupt them, and the rest of us tend to oblige. It is easy to listen to people who spend so much time researching their facts, and Ambers love facts.

SELF-DISCIPLINED

Ambers plan. They prepare. They produce. They achieve. They accomplish. And they do so systematically all throughout their lives. This amazing discipline serves Ambers in most areas of their lives, but it can fail them in one of the most important realms—that of relationships.

The thing for Ambers to remember in relationships with others is that people are more important than tasks. Ambers are so attached to their own plans and schedule that relationships get sacrificed in the name of goals and objectives. When Ambers are able to identify this blind spot, they become true pillars of excellence applying all their practiced self-discipline to people.

ACTS OF SERVICE

Ambers almost always show love through acts of service, especially when they prioritize people to the tops of their task lists and goals. Active service makes sense to Ambers. They can plan it, carry it out, and see it through to its useful consequences. In doing so, they show their best selves because they can once again apply discipline and repetition in service to others.

AMBER FAMOUS PEOPLE*

Jane Austen—writer
Charles Dickens—writer
Sean Connery—actor
Kelsey Grammar—actor
Tommy Lee Jones—actor
Martha Stewart—business magnate, producer & designer

Dale Earnhardt Jr. (Orange)—racecar driver
Charles Barkley (Orange)—professional basketball player, analyst & author
Thomas Newman (Magenta)—composer & conductor

*Parentheses signify the secondary part of their main Aura Personality.

~

AURA PERSONALITIES

THE GREEN AURA PERSONALITY

The Innovator

*"Green Days. Deep deep in the sea.
Cool and quiet fish. That's me."*
From *My Many Colored Day*s,
By Dr. Seuss

CALM, COOL, COLLECTED
Quiet, but not shy, Greens bring the rest of us down a notch, turning down the volume on overexcitement, over-anxiety and overreactions of any kind. Without realizing it, they are constantly emitting a "chill out"

vibe. They are uncomfortable with strong emotional responses in others and rarely manifest them themselves.

NONJUDGMENTAL SOUNDING BOARDS
Detached and laid back, Greens can be easy to talk to. They genuinely remain emotionally and mentally neutral in most situations. They just do not get caught up in emotional maelstrom or hype. Greens are true sounding boards by allowing others free exploration of their thoughts and feelings without judgment.

FAST, CONTINUAL LEARNERS
Bright and intelligent with quick, agile minds, Greens are ever interested in new things and ideas. The ability of their minds to chew on ideas and figure things out is staggering. They never tire of it. Sleep is their only break from it.

Greens choose whether or not they are interested in something, but once they decide they are, they learn everything they can about it with extreme speed. If they want to figure something out, they will. They learn best puzzling things out in their minds. Once they have figured something out, they move on quickly and abruptly.

UNLIMITED IN BUSINESS
Greens love business. It's a playground for their ideas, presenting countless mental challenges. Greens are often entrepreneurs because it allows them to create something that is currently of interest to them while at the same time providing constant new puzzles to solve. It's the ideal environment for the creative, problem-solving Greens. The business world knows no boundaries for ideas, products, and ways to expand

them, and their profitability. Greens are able to think as big as they want, without preconceived limitations others set upon themselves.

> *"If you're going to be thinking,
> you may as well think big."*
> Donald Trump

Business is a game for Greens, as is money, offering opportunities for strategizing and re-thinking. They get to put on their game face and work the system to their advantage. Greens like to be underestimated and keep others in the dark about their next move. These subtle power plays can be extremely advantageous in matters of money.

> *"It's always good to be underestimated."*
> Donald Trump

MONEY IS A PLAYTHING

Greens are shrewd and could keep themselves alive by their wits alone. They enjoy wheeling and dealing and getting stuff for free. They are clever and resourceful and don't experience money as a stressor like so many others do. Money is an ongoing game to be played. Greens may not always have it, but they can always find ways to get it.

Greens can waste time in their efforts to avoid paying for things. They like to figure out the system and avoid overpaying for anything. When others would not even think to, Greens will barter, get reduced prices, get reimbursed, or are given things for free. Stressful for others, this is play for Greens.

Green ♦ THE INNOVATOR

*"Money was never a big motivation for me,
except as a way to keep score.
The real excitement is playing the game."*
Donald Trump

Greens are almost always up for a challenge. They keep moving and plugging away at a scheme, a job, a strategy, a venture, undaunted by challenges and difficulties. They are optimists in this way, believing all will turn out well if they keep at it.

For all their thinking, they often solve problems through sudden insight or epiphanies. They have "ah-ha!" moments on a regular basis.

OPEN-MINDED, OUT-OF-THE-BOX THINKERS
The pot of thoughts, ever simmering with new ingredients, draws them in. No information is bad information. Greens will consider everything. They are extremely open-minded, out-of-the-box thinkers. It's that ability to consider all possibilities, all options, even the unorthodox ones, that allows for this alchemy to happen in an instant for them on a regular basis. Others call them fortunate, but this is the secret formula for their good fortune. Greens have the cool, silent confidence that the answers will come. They are patient, adaptable and flexible with the process and it rarely fails them.

STARTERS & INNOVATORS
Greens are starters; they possess the kind of optimism and courage that beginning anything requires. They are fearless to start new ventures and don't hesitate to step forward with their ideas. They don't even require capital, a plan, or support of others. They are greatly admired by others for this trait because it is uniquely theirs.

Greens are also innovators. Everything they touch, they find ways to improve. Technology is a fun playground for their minds because the possibilities and potential are endless.

UNDERRESPOND, UNDERREPLY, UNDERREACT

Greens are fearless in many ways. They have a tendency to under-respond and spend very little time in fear or worry. Their detached demeanor can minimize catastrophes.

Greens do not wallow in losses, even after calamities. They pick themselves up, brush themselves off, and start something new.

Their underresponsiveness can cause problems in relationships, especially for those who are external processors and need to speak with others in order to come to an understanding. It is important for Greens to realize this fundamental personality difference and being willing to respond, even with grunts, to confirm that they are listening to what the other person is saying.

UNDERESTIMATERS

Greens can underestimate things as well—like how long something will take, how much effort is required, or the danger of a particular situation. This can create unnecessary frustration for them and others but it has its benefits as well. Greens create calm around them because they generally assume that whatever everyone else is worrying about, will not be as bad as they think. Their presence neutralizes electrically overcharged emotional environments.

MAVERICKS

Greens are scientists, inventors, innovators, and mavericks. They are the true frontiersmen and women of all the personalities with their quick-draw stance, fierce independence, adaptability to all kinds of situations, and ability to roll with change. Greens are very selective about what they internalize, and they do not take on responsibilities that are not theirs. This gives them more mobility, freedom and flexibility to move ahead with their own ventures and adapt to change.

ADAPTIVE & NEED CONSTANT CHANGE

Greens don't necessarily see adapting to change as a skill because they love change. They seek it out when it is not already finding them. There are a few other personalities that also enjoy change, but none are as adept at integrating change and rising up to meet all of it's challenge as well as Greens.

Francois de la Rochefoucauld said, *"The only thing constant in life is change."* With the same absolution it may be said, *"The only thing constant in Greens is change!"* Change is ever-present for Greens. They seem to seek each other out. What appears like sudden, spontaneous change from a Green has probably been in the works for a while. They just forgot to mention it to anyone. Greens forget to mention a lot of things, so life with a Green can mean a lot of surprises, and a lot of change.

The quick minds of Greens need change. They perpetually crave new interests and ideas. Because they learn so rapidly when they are interested in a particular idea, Greens learn all they want and then move on to something new. This might appear as a short-attention span, but it is simply the learning style of a Green. They choose when they are interested in something, and for how long, and do not expend energy on things of no interest to them.

Greens practice a true economy of the mind. They do not fake interest in people or ideas if they have none. They cannot. Greens do not have any extra room in their minds to stew over irreconcilable differences.

Greens can lose interest quickly because they learn things and people so quickly. Relationships do not have much room to breathe or grow organically because Greens quickly decide they know all there is to know about others. They need to be conscious of this in relationships or they will not stay long with any one person. Greens have to consciously decide to stay and not be bored, and they have to remake those decisions often. They have to remind them selves that people serve a different role than other things they ponder.

TEACHERS
Greens fall into the role of teacher because of their love of ideas. They are life-long learners creating their own curriculum through hands-on experiences in risk-taking and life. They enjoy sharing those ideas with others. So the university setting can really suit them.

DETACHED & IN THEIR HEADS
Greens are oblivious to how detached they appear to everyone around them, lost in their own thoughts. They may even perceive themselves as conversationalists, and sometimes can be, but most things are just an interruption to the ongoing conversation in their own minds. Greens are so often busy working something out in their mind, daydreaming and creative problem solving;

that they often miss out on things happening right before their eyes.

Greens are similar to Lavenders in that they are both highly involved in the realm of thought, but while Lavenders are in the realm of visual imagery, Greens inhabit the land of ideas.

POKER-FACED
The most common expression on the face of Greens is a poker face. It makes them pretty difficult to read by others. They are a tough audience and others rarely know if they are interested, entertained, or bored. Greens do not give many outward cues of approval or interest, and others might feel constantly disappointed if they look to Greens for affirmation. Many of us tend to keep our reactions in check around Greens. For Greens, the world is full of people that overreact. Greens under-react and under-respond.

LOVE WORDS, NOT WORDINESS
To communicate effectively with Greens, remember that brevity is key. Greens love words, but not wordiness. They don't mince words themselves and are clever and thoughtful with the ones they choose. To Greens, words are a gift to be treated with respect. Wordiness and repetition are tiresome to Greens.

When Greens speak, they want their words remembered and valued. On the flip side, their brief words can be cutting in their concision, and they are not always aware of the effect their words have on others. Greens are very thick-skinned and have no idea how thin-skinned others can be at times.

A HARD AUDIENCE

People want acceptance from Greens, but their quiet, serious demeanor makes them seem unapproachable. Greens tend to fall into the role of stern, detached parent in many of their relationships. Their romantic partners might seek to fulfill childhood longing for acceptance with them, but will be left wanting. Greens do not play those roles for others. In fact, they run from codependency games.

WITTY PEACEGIVERS

That said, approval from Greens, goes a long way. Greens are witty, peaceful, and unassuming. They are unobtrusive and quiet in their living space. They do not ask much of others and do not expect much in return. The way to successful relationships with Greens is by accepting and the peace they bring. When they are no longer intimidated by their aloof nature, people begin to relish their consistently peaceful Green companions.

UNBIASED PRESENCE

Unlike many others, Greens can sometimes see things exactly as they are without superimposing any kind of agenda bias or emotion on a situation. They are able to act as truly unbiased, outside observers when necessary.

Greens have the ability to be absolutely present. They can dismiss all other thoughts, any emotions, and other people's agendas in order to be laser-focused on the issue at hand.

GREEN FAMOUS PEOPLE*
Albert Einstein—scientist
Bill Gates—entrepreneur
Donald Trump—entrepreneur
Anthony Hopkins—actor
Brad Pitt (Lavender)—actor
Dave Letterman—comedian & show host
Simon Cowell—entrepreneur & television producer
Anna Wintour (Violet)—editor-in-chief of Vogue
Kiefer Sutherland—actor
Colin Farrell—actor
Pierce Brosnan—actor
Gwyneth Paltrow (Green-Amber)—actor & singer
Michael Vartan (Crystal)—actor
Shrek

*Parentheses signify the secondary part of their main Aura Personality.

~

THE MENTAL-EMOTIONAL FAMILY
~

AURA PERSONALITIES

The Mental-Emotional Aura Personalities

The Mental-Emotional Aura Personalities take counsel from their heads but often follow their hearts. They strive for harmony between mind and heart.

They are logical, big-hearted people, quickly switching between these two ways of learning about and interacting with the world and with others. This can sometimes be confusing to those close to them. But the intentions of the Mental-Emotional Aura Personalities are always good. They never mean to harm or insult with the things they say or do. And relationships with them can be a great learning experience. The Mental-Emotional Aura Personalities recognize that life is a work-in-progress, which gives us all more breathing room to learn and grow.

The Mental-Emotional Aura Personalities are:

RED-AMBERS
BLUE- AMBERS

~

AURA PERSONALITIES

THE RED-AMBER
AURA PERSONALITY

The Storyteller

*"Storytellers are a threat. They threaten
all champions of control, they frighten usurpers
of the right-to-freedom of the human spirit."*
From *Anthills of the Savannah,* by Chinua Achebe

STORYTELLERS & BARDS
Picture an ancient hearth; campfire and assembly place of a nomadic tribe gathered in the darkness to relax and commune. Enter the Storyteller. The group becomes

silent, anticipating shock and amazement, delight and dismay, from the playful, unabashedly brazen gestures and phrases delivered by the exciting, unpredictable Master Teller-of-Tales.

Though the ancient teller is forgotten and long gone, the histories, traditions, religions and entire cultures he conjured and shaped persist, passing and changing from generation to generation by every new teller, and every new telling.

History can always boast those who bring us stories and entertainment. The stories they tell enrich our sense of place and purpose and teach us who we are and where we come from. They bring sense to chaos and help us psychologically integrate tragedy and other unexplainable life events.

> *"...Things as fragile as thought, a dream, a legend,*
> *they can go on and on.*
> *If you can change the way people think.*
> *The way they see themselves.*
> *The way they see the world.*
> *You can change the way people live their lives."*
> From *Choke*, by Chuck Palahnihk

More often than not, the very best storytellers are people with Red-Amber Aura Personalities. They inherit their role from their natural love of language, communication and interaction with people. Red-Ambers love people and love to be intimately involved with the human race as a whole. Red-Ambers marinate in society. They are extremely interesting people who are extremely interested in people.

NO SUBJECT IS OFF-LIMITS

Red-Ambers are very open. They are willing to share a lot about themselves in order to experience themselves, others and life more fully. What they share can sometimes make others uncomfortable because it can be more intimate or shocking than many of us are comfortable with. These boundaries fall outside the social comfort zone. They are accused of having no filter for what they discuss: no subject is off limits, and taboo topics are fair game.

One of the main reasons Red-Ambers say shocking things is to watch how people will respond. They are highly observant of verbal and nonverbal cues and use them to gather information about others.

> *"All the world's a stage."*
> William Shakespeare

PEOPLE & SOCIETY ARE THEIR SCHOOLING

Red-Ambers are fascinated with people. This fascination can easily roll into gossip and over-involvement in other peoples' lives. It can also cause problems with personal space. They do not seem to have a clear sense of personal space or of the personal physical boundaries of others.

Red-Ambers are so engaged, intrigued and involved with society it is like they are woven into its very fabric, experiencing every part of it. And, through their intimacy with all that is human—the good, the bad, the fantastical and mundane—they are able to accurately reflect us back to ourselves. This is one of the reasons that Red-Ambers feel a bit unsafe to some of us. They niggle us on the edge of our consciousness, revealing what we really are as a group.

OBJECTIVE OBSERVERS OF HUMAN NATURE

As close as they are to the group, Red-Ambers live just beyond the parameters of expected rules and customs. They do not hold fast to immediate moral codes because they are ever open to the possibility of something else. Red-Ambers are naturally impartial, which can appear somewhat amoral to others. In the interest of learning, they are testing boundaries, seeing how far they will stretch and by doing so, they learn about life and people. They are able to maintain the broader perspective that human nature is as it has always been, that it is not likely to change, and that some rules are simply customary with no intrinsic moral value.

BOUNDARY PUSHERS

That said, moral lines can become hazy for Red-Ambers, and they can become rule breakers, stretching the truth, if they are not careful. Red-Ambers can have too much pride in their own ideas and in their boundary-pushing behaviors, in particular. Obviously this can cause problems in many areas of their lives, especially their relationships. Because Red-Ambers tend to push negativity away, they can fail to see this, even when they are the cause.

LIFE IS A WORK-IN-PROGRESS

Red-Ambers do not like to admit fault and often see no need to change themselves. If they do admit their flaws or poor choices, it does not necessarily mean they believe they should change them. Part of the reason for this is that everything is a work-in-progress to Red-Ambers. If something is in question, then for them, it is probably not finished yet. They serve as constant reminders that we are ever transforming, ever-becoming.

RESOURCEFUL OUT-OF-THE-BOX THINKERS

The minds of Red-Ambers are like engineering contraptions, with weights and magnets, wheels and pulleys, generators and conveyer belts, simultaneously heading toward separate and particular conclusions. They are the out-of-the-box thinkers. The true Inventors, by every definition of the word, but especially as it applies to problem solving.

Scrappy and resourceful, there are absolutely no restrictions for how a problem might be approached or solved by Red-Ambers. With the rules thrown out, the realm of possibilities broadens considerably. Red-Ambers understand and utilize this principle better than anyone else. This ability alone makes them the most versatile and resourceful of all the personalities.

ARCHETYPAL TRICKSTER

Because so much about life is an open-ended question for Red-Ambers, they can be filled with doubt about themselves and others. Red-Ambers will feel confident about an idea, decision, or person one minute, and then change their mind the next. They can be tricky in relationships because they tend to trust and then withdraw trust often. They bring a push-pull dynamic to any relationship they are in. They can be fully vested and in the present one minute and then, in the next, they have switched into a distant, separate, even unhappy state.

Red-Ambers do a lot of switching and changing that leaves others reeling. They can be labeled the archetypal Trickster, stirring the pot, stoking the flame, causing unnecessary distractions. But, when all is said and done,

Red-Amber ♦ THE STORYTELLER

Red-Ambers mean well, and Tricksters do not. At the core of Red-Ambers is a very big, generous heart

MULTIPLE, ONGOING THOUGHT PATTERNS
One of the most important traits to understand about Red-Ambers is their complex thought patterns. They have many thoughts simultaneously and can rapidly move between those thoughts. This is reflected most clearly in their speech. Red-Ambers speak rapidly and tend to jump from topic to topic without finishing sentences or completing ideas aloud. As a result, they are often misunderstood. This is a source of great frustration for them.

ABSENT-MINDED PROFESSOR
They personify the absent-minded professor in many ways. With so much going on in their minds and so many and varied activities going on in their lives, Red-Ambers can appear very disconnected in conversation. They have to consciously concentrate to stay with the concept the other person is communicating, as well as disregard all the new thoughts rapidly flashing within their own minds.

EXCITING, SURPRISING & INTERESTING
On the other hand, Red-Ambers make very interesting companions because you never know what you are going to get from them. Their communication style and the way they think make them exciting and varied friends, companions and storytellers. There is never a dull moment around Red-Ambers. The way they think and operate is like watching a natural phenomenon at the peak of activity.

VERSATILE

Red-Ambers manage many activities at once. They are difficult to track for all their thinking, plotting and involvement. They are able to start something new right in the middle of another unfinished task. To others, the life of a Red-Amber looks like multiple whirlwinds of random activity.

All of this activity creates stress and worry for themselves and others. It also encourages forgetfulness. A balanced and organized life is a challenge for Red-Ambers. In particular, they have to watch pack-rat tendencies. They can fill their minds and their lives with clutter if they are not mindful of this. With the speed and variety of their thoughts and activities, it is no surprise that Red-Ambers get frazzled, harried, touchy, and are sometimes verbally attacking when overloaded.

Red-Ambers need to take great care not to burn out mentally and physically. Exercise, good nutrition and spiritual rituals-all unnatural routines for Red-Ambers-can bring tremendous balance to their lives.

JACKS-&-JILLS-OF-ALL-TRADES

One gift of these incredibly versatile people is their ability to try on various roles, and take on many responsibilities. They are the Jacks-and-Jills-of-all-trades. Throughout their lives they find they are suited to just about anything for a time, something that just is not the case for any other personality.

POLITICIANS

One role that particularly suits Red-Ambers is that of politician. Red-Ambers are more than equipped to handle the independent and versatile lifestyles of politicians. Politics utilize many of their innate gifts, including their ability to captivate audiences with their charm and candor. Red-Ambers are fast talkers and walkers and can keep the fast pace and long hours a political life requires. They have a strong sense of their own capability and are able to convince others of the same.

Red-Ambers can juggle many tasks and a great number of relationships simultaneously. Even the limited term in office suits their need for change and the loss of stamina they experience when they are ready to engage elsewhere. It would be no surprise to find, in days past, that many royal court jesters were also secret political advisors. One recent example of a Red-Amber in a political role is former president of the United States, George W. Bush.

WARM-HEARTED
Although politics suit them, it is only one of a multitude of hats Red-Ambers might wear throughout their lives. They are as interesting and eclectic as the myriad of things they collect in their homes.

Red-Ambers are colorful, animated, charming, fun, happy, flirty, vibrant, complimentary and persistent people. They have a constant twinkle in their eye, an engaging story to tell and a happy countenance to spread nearly all of the time.

Red-Ambers exude warmth and can be very engaging, when they choose to be. They are sensitive individuals. This means they are tender and loving, but it also means they can be easily offended. They are situationally thick-skinned—can dish it, but cannot always take it in return.

Nonetheless, all ill will can be un-done for Red-Ambers with sincere praise. Words go far with these verbose folk.

> *I need to be praised
> almost as much as I need to be liked.*
> Michael Scott, *The Office*

EASILY OFFENDED
Red-Ambers tend to take personal offense even for things that are not personal. In fact, they are probably the most easily offended Aura-Personality. Part of this is due to the fact that they are such socially involved people. Red-Ambers have the ability to get involved with people. They easily join many social circles that, in turn, expose them to a lot of relationship drama. Things not personal to most become personal to them within these circles.

Because they feel it is such a great risk to open their hearts to others, if someone lets them down, they can hold onto offenses for a long time. Red-Ambers have a tendency to really feel let down when others disappoint them or do not meet their standards.

GENEROUS
Praise them and they will work to please you. Red-Ambers are generous by nature—generous in praise, generous in hospitality, generous in giving and in service, when they decide to be. They do many kind things for others, on their own terms; these acts can seem sudden and random to the other person.

Red-Ambers have their hearts in the right place. They need to please others, and they need to be liked (even more than they need to be praised). So if you let them know you like them, are grateful for them, and praise them, they will soar in confidence and exude kindness.

RED-AMBER FAMOUS PEOPLE*
Oprah Winfrey—talk show host & entrepreneur
Ellen DeGeneres—talk show host & comedian
Steve Carell (Green)—actor
Carol Burnett (Yellow)—comedian, singer, dancer & writer
Shahruhk Khan—Bollywood actor
George W. Bush—former U.S. president
Jack Hanna—naturalist
Wolfgang Puck—chef & restaurateur

*Parentheses signify the secondary part of their main Aura Personality.

~

AURA PERSONALITIES

THE BLUE-AMBER AURA PERSONALITY

The Ministering Angel

> *"Give your hands to serve and your hearts to love."*
> — Mother Teresa

TIRELESS IN RENDERING SERVICE

Helping others with acts of kindness and thinking of ways to help (when they are not actually in the act of serving) are the mode of operation for Blue-Ambers. They are seemingly tireless in their acts of charity. It is astounding for the rest of us to see just how tireless they are. It is a single-focused, constant, high-physical-output way of serving. It is the loaves of bread left on doorsteps, spending their vacation time helping someone else pack and move, and leaving notes of encouragement. There are too many ways to mention how Blue-Ambers serve others. But a good sampling can be found in the New Testament, performed by Jesus and his disciples.

Blue-Ambers constantly invent new ways to serve. Where there is a need, Blue-Ambers find a way to help; that is the purpose of their being, their joy in life. Nothing brings Blue-Ambers a greater sense of fulfillment than serving others in need.

REGAL SERVANTS
Blue-Ambers are educated people, formally or informally, and raise the bar of refinement for everyone else. They are drawn to what is proper and genteel. They are well-mannered, soft spoken and tactful in all they say and do.

Blue-Ambers are naturally elegant, classy and regal. Unaware of this, they carry an air of nobility coupled with humility that is so sweet and beautiful. They instill a sense of dignity in others by association, and they are dignified even while wearing blue jeans and emptying bedpans. Blue-Ambers pass on class to those around them. They ennoble us.

GRACIOUS & GENEROUS
Even though they are soft spoken, Blue-Ambers never hold back compliments. They pour verbal praise onto others. Although they do appreciate and need gratitude for all their tireless charity, they are more concerned with extending it to others. They are very gracious, always verbally acknowledging any kindness extended to them.

*Kindness in words
creates confidence.
Kindness in thinking
creates profoundness.
Kindness in giving
creates love."*
Lao Tzu

SELF-EFFACING

Interestingly, for all the praise they lavish on others, Blue-Ambers are very self-effacing. They are uncomfortable with the spotlight and quickly redirect it to someone else if it is shined on them.

Blue-Ambers tend to deflect all compliments and praise; they need to be careful with this trait-a lot of negative words come out when they are referring to themselves. Blue-Ambers are natural role models for so many people, so this is an important trait to acknowledge and eliminate. Blue-Ambers can learn to accept praise and compliments; in doing so, they give others the same permission.

Blue-Ambers can use their self-abnegation as a way to make others feel comfortable. They feel adoration from others, but they tend to want to deflect it away from themselves. They do this through self-effacing humor that is often quite funny, but they need to take care not to use too much negativity with their wit.

NONDISCRIMINATING

Blue-Ambers are undiscriminating in service. No one falls outside their reach for kindness, or outside the realm of worthiness to be assisted by them.

> *"Let us touch the dying, the poor, the lonely and the unwanted according to the graces we have received and let us not be ashamed or slow to do the humble work."*
> Mother Teresa

Blue-Ambers are all-inclusive. The phrase *No one left behind* is a mantra they live from more than anyone else. They are not racist, ageist or sexist. All are equal in their eyes. All are deserving of love and care. Their large circle of friends reflects this—nearly everyone they meet becomes a friend.

Blue-Ambers are too busy serving the person with the greatest need to hangout with friends or spend time with any one person for long. They maintain friendships with kind words and deeds, and they invite everyone to everything. They will single-handedly make sure you feel welcome and included.

BRING OUT THE BEST IN OTHERS
Because we really look up to Blue-Ambers, and admire their goodness, we feel it a special privilege to be called their friends. Blue-Ambers make you feel like you are really important because, to them, you are! They literally affect the core self-esteem of everyone they encounter. We think, "Well, if they like me, and I make them smile, I must be important, likeable and worthwhile."

Every one feels more self-dignity in the presence of Blue-Ambers. No one is beyond a Blue-Amber's belief in them. Your intrinsic value is crystal clear to them. So, inevitably, it is magnified in their presence. You feel of worth. Your worth becomes self-evident in their presence.

Blue-Ambers bring out the gentler, more loving side in all of us. We all like ourselves better in their presence. We take more care over what we say and do around them. It is hard not to respect them because they so naturally garner respect with their deeds and demeanor, and we want to be more good and kind because of their goodness and kindness.

ACCOMMODATING & CODEPENDENT
Blue-Ambers almost always have the intention of helping and acceptance in all of their interactions and relationships. This altruistic stance leaves them understandably vulnerable because others can take them for granted and take advantage of them. Blue-Ambers can be so allowing of others' weaknesses that they actually enable negative behavior; in this way, their open acceptance of others can backfire.

Some reasons Blue-Ambers often tolerate inappropriate behavior are: to keep the peace, and to help others feel better about themselves. Blue-Ambers try to make up the difference of other people's lack—which is not their job. This tendency falls within the bounds of codependency and is called "enablement." It is inappropriate behavior, but difficult for Blue-Ambers to see in themselves. After all, their intention is to help, and their primary focus is to have others know they are accepted and acceptable, unconditionally.

There is a balance that needs to be reached with regards to appropriate boundaries. Blue-Ambers can and do learn these boundaries over time, but unfortunately, it often happens the hard way, through force, when someone takes advantage of their kindness.

SENTIMENTAL & HOMEY

Blue-Ambers are sentimental. They notice even the smallest acts of kindness others do. They like to receive and give gifts that have personal significance. They add a personal touch to everything they create and they appreciate the same from others.

Blue-Amber homes are adorned in things children and friends make for them. They have homes that are personal and personable. They want everyone around them to feel peace, safety and comfort.

SUPPORTING ROLE

Blue-Ambers are very supportive of others. They support and actively encourage the talents and gifts of others. They do this by attending events, keeping records, giving lots of praise, and making sacrifices to help people further their interests and talents. Once again, it is nice if Blue-Ambers can extend such kindness and encouragement to themselves, and to their own talents and abilities.

IMPOSE OWN STANDARD ON OTHERS

Blue-Ambers feel the needs of others so deeply, and the instinct to give physical assistance and take action is so acute that it is difficult for them to imagine any other way of giving. Because of this, they tend to impose their moral code onto others, believing all of us should respond to situations and to the needs of others the way they do.

There are countless other ways to give service to others. Sometimes it is difficult to remember this, for them and for us, because acts of service are the most obvious way; the most visible, external, and acknowledged. Blue-

Ambers are immediate in the way they give help; sometimes they may not consider that a person's needs may be different. We all have different things we need to contribute to this world and each other. Charity is a much-valued offering from Blue-Ambers; each Aura Personalities offerings are uniquely valuable, in their own distinctive way.

Blue-Ambers often make the mistake of assuming that others will find the same character building results and satisfaction from serving. But it is not the same for others. In fact, loved ones can begin to resent serving in that capacity. They can feel like beasts of burden, used for their ability to labor, instead of being allowed to give to the world their particular brand of service.

Blue-Ambers need to make sure they don't guilt or coax those around them to do as they do, in terms of service. The level of doing-ness of a Blue-Amber is well beyond the limits of any other personality, although Ambers run a close second. So expecting or requiring others to get on board with all of their projects and missions can be very taxing and stressful for their children, spouses, and friends, certain personalities more than others.

Interestingly, if Blue-Ambers knew they were creating discord, or limiting others in any way, they would immediately change their outlook. Blue-Ambers are our best cheerleaders. Whatever we are good at, they will champion us more than anyone else.

SERVICE CAN LIMIT CLOSENESS TO OTHERS
While Blue-Ambers are busy blessing the lives of the needy, their friends and family are looking for ways to get closer to them. Many of them will enlist in Blue-

Amber service projects and missions in order to create emotional closeness.

Blue-Ambers are introverted and private, and because of their constant do good mode of operating, they can often seem quite remote and unavailable to those closest to them. It is hard for them to stop doing and just spend time with or hang out with their loved ones. This is because it feels lazy and unproductive to them. They have a constant nagging inside them telling them that someone needs their service, so they feel they cannot afford to be idle. But sometimes, the service needed from them the most is to relax, play and have fun with those closest to them.

FUTURE-ORIENTED
Blue-Ambers like to be in the know. They keep themselves abreast of situations and events to avoid being left in the dark. They like to know what to expect and plan their lives accordingly.

Relaxing is easier said than done for Blue-Ambers. They are future-oriented; always considering what is next on the agenda; perpetually looking and moving forward. Blue-Ambers are doers second only to Ambers. They also share Amber traits of stress, having high performance expectations of themselves and others, and worrying about what is next instead of focusing on the present moment.

OVERLY SELF-SUFFICIENT
For all that they offer others, Blue-Ambers have difficulty accepting help from others. They are extremely self-sufficient, to the point that they can be doing things for others almost all of the time. If they are not aware of

this, they can become prideful in this way. But they need help too, and it is important for them to allow others the opportunity to serve.

NEED FOR BALANCE
Blue-Ambers are so naturally thoughtless of themselves, and thoughtful of others, that they often allow their health to decline, gradually, but constantly. They literally *wear their lives away in the service of others*, as the saying goes. But Blue-Ambers do not want to be worn out. They want to be useful. Devoting discipline toward self-care is a skill they have to acquire.

Blue-Ambers have a hard time making their needs known to others. Similar to Blues, Lavenders and Crystals, Blue-Ambers take the victim-like position assuming others will meet their needs without having to ask. Part of the reason for this tendency is that they are all people who are watching closely to see how they can meet the unspoken needs of others. This is a beautiful trait, but it also borders on irresponsibility. We are all responsible for creating balance in our own lives.

SEE INJUSTICE & FEEL VICTIMHOOD
Blue-Ambers are very unhappy that injustice exists, both for themselves and others. They feel victimized by it and believe that bad things should not happen to anyone.

Blue-Ambers would have the world be a kind, safe haven for all. They believe in and hope for a fairytale world (and can often be disillusioned by reality), similar to Blues. This can transition them into depression, helplessness or hopelessness, if they are not watchful. It is part of the reason they keep moving, performing nonstop acts of kindness, individual by individual. It is their way of holding back the tide of doom that so easily crowds in when we are not watching.

NEGATIVITY CAN BLINDSIDE THEM

Blue-Ambers have to guard against taking offense and being disappointed by the action or inaction of others. If they are not careful, they can down-spiral in feeling let down.

Blue-Ambers need to let go of grudges and forget past offenses. They have to work on their tendency to take things personally just as Red-Ambers do. They erroneously believe that they are expressing compassion by holding tightly to offenses and will do far more good by letting them go.

When Blue-Ambers get buried in negative storylines, (their own or someone else's) they can carry it around like a brick, sharing too much negativity with others, getting short-sighted within the emotional aspect of the story, and feeling helpless to change it. They frequently vacillate between empowerment and victimhood as a result of injustices and being able to separate from them.

Despite this, Blue-Ambers keep moving and serving because they never forget that someone else is suffering more than they are. They would have more energy for their service, however, if they would allow themselves to emotionally let go of the negativity.

> *"The best revenge is living well."*
> Jerry Seinfeld

HOLD BACK TIDE OF UNFAIRNESS WITH HUMANITARIAN SERVICE

Blue-Ambers bandwagon for change and show the world how we can help dissolve injustice and inhumanity. They call upon our higher senses, petition our wallets, and then they get down into the trenches and make positive change happen.

> *"Do not wait for leaders;
> do it alone, person to person."*
> Mother Teresa

DIPLOMATIC DARK HORSE

Blue-Ambers are working in nonprofits and humanitarian organizations the world over. They are extending kindness and creating respect between countries and governments.

Blue-Ambers can help smooth over uncomfortable situations and get through political doors that others see as permanently shut. They are natural diplomats and we are wise to use them in such roles. It is difficult to refuse people who follow through with their word without asking anything in return. Blue-Ambers are quietly powerful, expanding minds and opening hearts through their kindness and tireless service.

> *"Compassion is not a religious business,
> it is a human business,
> it is not a luxury, it is essential
> for our own peace and mental stability,
> it is essential for survival."*
> Dalai Lama

BLUE-AMBER FAMOUS PEOPLE*
Mother Teresa—humanitarian
Paul Newman—actor & philanthropist
Jerry Seinfeld (Lavender)—comedian, actor, writer & television producer
Brian Regan (Yellow)—comedian
Jewel (Lavender)—singer & songwriter
Tom Hanks (Yellow)—actor & equal rights advocate
Sally Fields—actor
Shel Silverstein—author

*Parentheses signify the secondary part of their main Aura Personality.

AURA PERSONALITIES

THE EMOTIONAL FAMILY

~

AURA PERSONALITIES

The Emotional Aura Personality Family

The Emotional Aura Personality Family is a family of one, but that one has such a big heart it can hold all the other Aura Personalities combined. Though it can be to their detriment at times, being "all heart" is an amazing ability.

Those who are in the Emotional Aura personality Family have highly attuned emotional systems. They experience the world and others primarily through emotions, and they teach the rest of us to tune into what our emotions are telling us. They demonstrate what full emotional expression means, and have the highest potential for emotional intelligence.

The Emotional Aura Personalities are:

BLUES

~

THE BLUE AURA PERSONALITY

The Heart Guardian

> *"I'm convinced that the biggest human blockage is the unwillingness to fully experience the intensity of our emotions."*
> From *Quantum Touch*,
> By Richard Gordon

Enormous hearts are the defining characteristic of people with Blue Aura Personalities—hearts far too large to be contained within a single person. Blues bear this heavy burden willingly as a generous gesture of love for the rest of us. They are willing to care for the emotional well being of our world, day-by-day, loving and nurturing the people in their lives.

EMOTIONAL RISK-TAKERS
Blues live from a more purely emotional place than any other aura personality. They are the emotional risk-takers and are here to help the rest of us experience our feelings more deeply, fully and truthfully.

Try as they might, Blues cannot contain their emotions, nor should they try. Suppressing their emotions would feel like holding their breath underwater too long. However, if they do not perceive emotional expression as safe or welcome, that is exactly what they figuratively do. They sink into despondency, and feel that their lungs might burst and their hearts might break. Lucky for us, Blues are naturally tenacious. They are survivors that will willfully increase their lung capacity over time and stitch back together their highly intelligent hearts. Blues at peace with the emotional world, which is as big and deep as the sea, are anchors for all of us as we navigate this emotionally charged experience called life.

Judged since childhood for being overly emotional or too sensitive, Blues face much criticism, and even mockery, for trusting fiercely in their hearts. But critics should beware. Using their hearts as compasses is their precious gift to us. Blues are a barometer of love for the whole world, without which we would be barren and lost, leading emotionally isolative lives.

HEALING HEARTS
Because of the general disdain in our culture for overt displays of emotion, Blues have learned to suppress, or

become overly logical, about what is an otherwise innate knowing. That *knowing* is their gift. At their core, Blues know that our collective heart can heal the planet, but they have to accept their own hearts before they can awaken others.

ANTENNAE FOR EMOTIONAL FREQUENCIES

Blues are the antennae for all emotional frequencies—yours, mine, and their own. Their emotions are their primary brain centers, from which they gather data, choose their responses, and navigate through most areas of life. In fact, Blues might be tempted to define the whole world by their emotional response to it.

BORN PSYCHOLOGISTS & COUNSELORS

Blues extreme sensitivity to emotional undercurrents has been a highly undervalued talent, until the recent emergence of psychotherapy in the mid-twentieth century. The field of Psychology continually serves as a repository for Blue interpersonal and relational gifts, where Blues have been able to define and refine the human emotional and psychological experience, even birthing a common language for the heart.

GUARDIANS OF RELATIONSHIPS

Although Blues jump into causes-like psychology and human rights-as a place to funnel all the emotional intensity of love they feel, their focus is always and primarily, on relationships. Blues are the natural guardians of relationships. They think in terms of relationships, they are happiest inside of loving, romantic and familial relationships, and they rarely consider themselves separate or apart from relationships.

RELATIONSHIPS ARE THEIR SCHOOLING

There is no place Blues will learn more about themselves and others than inside relationships, nor is there any place they would rather learn. Blues will travel great emotional and physical distances to help relationships. They will leave comfort and routine behind if they believe it will strengthen that bond. All of their greatest risks are in the name of relationships. Within relationships they uncover their innate gifts, interpersonal skills, and tremendous capacity for sympathy, care, concern, compassion and love.

CODEPENDENCY CYCLE

With such enormous hearts, Blues cannot help feeling enormous obligation within the relationship context. The major stumbling block for them is that, as they sort out these roles and responsibilities, they easily stumble into codependency; their greatest weakness lies at the heart of their greatest gift. However, if they will take responsibility for it, that gift will greatly benefit all of us.

MISDIRECTED CARETAKING

In the strict psychological definition of the word, codependent Blues are hooked into the emotional climate around them, to the point that they cannot always find the way out. They have difficulty adjusting the volume of the emotional data pouring in. As a result, they often have a hard time separating out where they end and others begin. Blues naturally inhabit all the classic characteristics of caretakers, in codependency terminology.

One caretaking trait Blues carry, (along with other Aura Personalities that have spiritual or emotional energy), is that of being a pleaser. Pleasers "make nice" as an indirect method for controlling the emotional climate in relationships. They over-compliment. This is a means of focusing attention on others in order to divert it away from themselves. They do not like feeling that they are the cause of an upset, nor do they like having someone upset with them, so they might manifest a false positive emotion in order to curtail or avoid awkwardness, or any other strong negative reaction or emotion. They might try to work through their own complicated emotions by showing up in the therapist or friend role for others, using that setting as an indirect means for getting their own emotional needs met. This last behavior will feel uncomfortable to others, but they may not be able to define why that is.

Blues often assume they know what others are feeling, needing or wanting. This can be frustrating for others because, in their assumptions Blues can miss the bigger picture that others would like to explore and understand. Emotions are not the only factor many of us consider when we are sorting through the complications of life, so Blue views can sometimes feel narrow.

MISUSE OF EMOTIONAL INTIMACY
There is a learning curve for Blues as they help others explore emotions, but if they are not careful and respectful in the unveiling, others end up feeling emotionally exposed instead.

A characteristic of Blues, in particular, is misusing their great talent for intimacy as a means to get others to share feelings, before they are ready to share. Since most people are extremely private with their emotional lives, emotional probing can feel invasive and uncomfortable. It is one of their greatest gifts but, if misused, it can also be a source of their greatest pain, separating them from those closest to them. Blues have to practice respect and self-control when they are giving counsel or support to others. Appropriate boundaries are essential for them to be effective in matters of the heart.

INDIRECT

All of us share some responsibility for Blues inability to see their unhealthy, codependent and caretaking tendencies. We are to partly to blame because we so often mislabel unhealthy Blue behavior as sweet and Blue people as "the nicest people ever." While these may be true statements, they can also be veiled ways of avoiding dealing with all the indirect, uncomfortable, invasive energy that comes with all that niceness. There is truth to these statements but, underneath, lies an inability to admit that we are uncomfortable with the emotional boundaries of Blues; that we are unwilling to be direct and responsible for our own emotions. Through our mutual indirectness, we create separation and pain in our relationships with them.

RELATIONSHIPS ARE THEIR PLAYGROUND

The boundaries of relationships and their accompanying emotions are like a natural playground for Blues. Because Blues are constantly asking all the right questions about relationships, in order to overcome their native weakness in this area, they have all the best answers to these boundaries-in-relationships questions.

If Blues will allow themselves to see their tendencies towards codependency and caretaking, they will begin to effortlessly weave straw into gold with their knowledge. They will purify their heart and create a clean, honest, rich and beautiful emotional world for us to inhabit, both symbiotically and separately.

Although other aura personality types might have tendencies toward codependency, Blues will ultimately reveal its demise as they unravel the heart from codependency constraints and shift it into the freedom and expansion of interdependent relationships.

> *"Among the blessings of love*
> *there is hardly one more exquisite*
> *than the sense that uniting the beloved life to ours*
> *we can watch over its happiness,*
> *bring comfort where hardship was,*
> *and over memories of privation and suffering*
> *open the sweetest fountains of joy."*
> From Daniel Deronda, By George Eliot

NURTURERS

Blues wish everything in the world were softer, lovelier, friendlier, and kinder. They nurture us and remind us of our own stewardship; to love and care for one another while we are together on this planet.

Blues cannot relate to sharp words or mean glances. Unkindness is baffling and painful to their tender hearts. So, as you interact with Blues, be kinder than you naturally would with your words, your touch, and your ways. There is a need in the world to tone down our harshness and carelessness and create more beauty in its place.

HOPELESS ROMANTICS

Not surprisingly, as guardians of the heart, Blues are also the stewards of romance and fantasy. Blues imagine a magical, beautiful, romance-filled world but they can often feel let down when their reality falls short of their limitless imaginings.

Blues are the hopeless romantics. They often fall within the "If Only" group: If only this would change, then I would be happy; If this person would like me, then I would be happy; If this person did this for me, then my needs would be met. As part of their boundaries-in-relationships learning process, Blues must avoid too easily handing over their happiness to others. They feel so much vibrancy within their own hearts that they are often surprised not to find it in the external world and feel deeply let down by life. Somehow, despite constant disappointment, they remain hopeful that the fairytale is still out there, somewhere. They are tenacious, even in this.

The danger is that if the fairytale is "out there," then it's probably not "right here" in front of them. Blues have a tendency to see disappointment in the present and something better as yet to come. For Blues, that something better often appears in the form of a rescuer, to save the damsel or prince-in-distress. Their struggle is in accepting that fairy tale elements can occur in their everyday life.

PEDESTALLING & BEING LET DOWN

Blues often place others on pedestals where the only direction left to travel is down. With the kindest of intentions, Blues have a powerful desire to see everyone and everything as extraordinary. We all "fall from grace" easily; no one can live up to the fairytale image created by another.

The idea behind this is that someone else is responsible for his or her happiness. This can become yet another game of codependency Blues create and is an important dynamic to identify about the way they experience the world and other people.

BRING ROMANCE & MAGIC TO THE WORLD

When all is said and done, there is a wonderful understanding that comes from this natural tendency to feel like a wounded character from a fairy tale world. Through this, Blues come to realize, consciously or not, that if the world is not going to bring the magical kingdom to their doorstep, then they are going to create it and bring it to the world.

From somewhere deep within, Blues begin to build a magnificent world, brick-by-brick, beauty-by-beauty, through extremely creative means. They begin to create, for themselves and the rest of us, what they knew was possible but were unable to find until they looked within. And, if they can extend their grace to others long enough to create these extraordinary worlds, we all get to be extraordinary in them together.

COLOR THE WORLD WITH RICHNESS

Blues naturally desire and imagine the fantastical, and can make everything better than reality by creating what they desire. More than anyone else, they have the ability to manifest the fairytale with knights and princesses, swords, glory, royalty, romance, intrigue, soft fabrics, fine furnishings, luxuriant flavors and smells, fine culture, and decadence in both beauty and pleasure.

Blues are writing, making and creating, in organizations and in homes, infusing all of our lives with richness. The world is an infinitely more beautiful place because Blues share our planet.

HIGHLY SENSUAL
With beauty comes comfort and sensuality. Blues are very naturally sensual. They long to be desired and place a priority on making themselves desirable to others. In relationships with Blues, they can surprise you with bold emotional and sensual gestures or statements. They reign supreme in the realm of romance in relationships; their confidence is made clear through their sensuality.

SENTIMENTAL & UNSURE
On the offset, they are emotionally tender, hesitant and unsure with others and can struggle with feeling unimportant, undervalued or unappreciated. They are sentimental, so what you say or give means something to them. Blues can be naïve and always like to make sure everyone else is comfortable; the rest of us should not take advantage of this trait. They spend a lot of energy keeping things upbeat in an effort to smooth out the roughness of this stark world. Instead of teasing them for it, the rest of us can choose to add to all the beauty they are already creating.

POTENTIAL FOR TRUE INTIMACY
One of the downfalls to their sometimes-forced cheeriness is that it does not allow for a full range of emotions in others or in them. More than anything, Blues desire the kind of deep emotional connection that kind of sharing would evoke. If others don't have to worry about stepping on Blue toes, then there will be much more possibility for true intimacy. Blues desire true intimacy more than anything else and, if they have

it, they are ecstatic beings that the rest of us are so lucky to know.

GIVE THOUGHTFULNESS ONE-BY-ONE
Relationships are at the center of Blue lives and their purpose for being; they need to be recognized and valued for all of the kind, thoughtful things they do and say to create a happy, fun, comfortable environment for everyone. Because they do so much for others, it is preferable for them to be in clearly defined roles within all of their relationships where they can show that concern and care one-on-one.

HIGH EMOTIONAL INTELLIGENCE
There is a scene in Snow White & The Seven Dwarves when the dwarves find Snow White sleeping in their cottage. When Snow White awakens, she knows the name of each dwarf immediately, based on expressions and posturing. The dwarves' names are all based on emotions and Snow White has no problem distinguishing one emotion from another.

Such is the emotional intelligence of Blues. They can readily detect the emotions of anyone in their vicinity. The emotional input they receive from others is very loud. It can be exhausting for them to channel so much emotional information. For Blues, the emotional information is the most important and it is difficult for them not to see it as the sum total of what is going on with a person. But other factors may be equally or even more weighty for others.

The heart is their compass and barometer as they navigate through life and relationships. Blues trust their hearts above all else and it hurts them when the emotional information they bring to the forefront is discounted. Blues will continue to prompt the rest of us to examine our heart and be aware of our emotions. This is one of their greatest services to us.

ENCOURAGEMENT & SELF-CARE
Blues encourage and compliment others, and thrive if both are lavished upon them as well. They enjoy giving and receiving nice things, as well as creating and experiencing nice environments. They are willing to make sacrifices in order to create both.

Luckily for them, Blues do self-care, pampering and "guilty pleasures" really well. Unlucky for them, indulgent food can serve as false comfort and they can fall easily into emotional-eating habits. If they are clear about this tendency, they can keep it in check by adding variety to the kinds of comfort, goodness and sweetness they bring into their lives.

CELEBRATIONS & TRADITIONS
Blues experience great satisfaction in planning and participating in celebrations; particularly all the significant emotional landmarks, like birthdays, weddings, anniversaries, reunions and even funerals. Blues love to spotlight people on an individual basis. They go to great lengths to make sure a celebration is tailor-made for the individual. And they are willing to do this for children, spouses, relatives, close friends, and even casual acquaintances. It is part of the way they show that each person, with their individual personalities, likes, dislikes, talents and uniqueness, deserves all of the limelight once in awhile.

These celebratory occasions are one way the rest of us can show Blues their value to us. Though we can give generous words of gratitude for all they do for us, we can also make these days in their lives really special. These celebrations are a way we can provide them a way to live out their fantasies in real life and let them be king or queen for a day. They deserve it after all they do to create the fairytale world for the rest of us so often.

BLUE FAMOUS PEOPLE*
Carl Heinrich Bloch—19th century Danish painter
Vincent Van Gogh (Lavender)—19th century Dutch painter
Grace Coddington (Lavender)—Creative Director of Vogue
Karen Grassle (Green-Amber)—actor
Mandy Moore—actor & singer
Drew Barrymore—actor & producer
Ann Hathaway—actor
Mira Sorvino—actor
Amy Adams—actor, singer & dancer

Pepé Le Pew
Snow White

*Parentheses signify the secondary part of their main Aura Personality.

~

THE EMOTIONAL-SPIRITUAL FAMILY
~

AURA PERSONALITIES

The Emotional-Spiritual Aura Personalities

The Emotional-Spiritual Aura Personalities have high emotional intelligence and strong intuitive abilities. Their intuition creates some emotional distance so they can objectively observe the emotional climate of any situation.

Ever watchful, the Emotional-Spiritual Aura Personalities experience and understand the world through both emotional and intuitive faculties. They are able to know things about us that help us on our individual and collective journeys.

The Emotional-Spiritual Aura Personalities are:

VIOLETS
LAVENDERS

~

AURA PERSONALITIES

THE VIOLET
AURA PERSONALITY

The Influencer

"The price of greatness is responsibility."
Winston Churchill

BORN LEADERS

Violets are the born leaders of this world. They may not always hold positions of high public profile, but they are always influencing a wide range of people at any given time.

Adaptable, assertive and strong, Violets continually keep the wheels of society turning. They do not know what it means to be stuck. They make things happen and, like Winston Churchill's call-to-action against Hitler during World War II; the things they make happen are often life altering. Violets do not know how to do anything small. Maybe the change they create is not always global, but it is always big.

PERSUASIVE MOTIVATORS

With their powers of persuasion, Violets get others up and moving. They never accept defeat, nor do they tolerate anyone else wallowing in it. Instead, they push us through defeat and towards reform. Their influence moves us toward broader ways of thinking and operating. Violets adapt to and implement new ideas quickly.

PROACTIVE PROBLEM-SOLVERS

Violets are brilliant individuals with busy minds, who are constantly innovating and seeing how to do things better. Their ability to solve complex problems at home, at work, or anywhere else is staggering. Their minds flip through a rapid succession of scenarios until they arrive at what they see as the most comprehensive solution; there is barely time for an intake of breath before that solution is implemented.

TRADITIONALISTS & VISIONARIES

Violets prefer to be viewed as traditionalists, but there is no mistaking the revolutionary spirit they harbor. They value and utilize both the wisdom of the past as well as the possibilities of the future for dealing with present issues.

> *"A love of tradition*
> *has never weakened a nation,*
> *indeed it has strengthened nations*
> *in their hour of peril;*
> *but the new view must come,*
> *the world must roll forward."*
> Winston Churchill

Violets seem to innately understand when to hold fast to a tradition and when to let it go. They never go against tradition in haste, as they have great respect for and learn much from, the past. Though they remind us often to look to the past for its universal lessons, Violets are also forward-thinkers. They are in sync with the shifting of our planet; they often serve as the catalysts-socially, politically and spiritually. If change is needed for us to progress, Violets will push it into being without hesitation.

> *"The further back I look,*
> *the further forward I can see."*
> Winston Churchill

INNATELY INTELLIGENT

Violets are highly intelligent, brilliant individuals that affect the world in big ways regardless of their level of formal education. They are born with the ability to gather knowledge anywhere and are innately street smart. With both of those gifts, they are ever conceptualizing and formulating answers and solutions. Violets think they are right most of the time and, since they consider a far greater number of factors in any given situation than most people, they often are.

INTERNALLY DRIVEN WITH HIGH MORALS
When Violets do share solutions or opinions, there is no subtlety involved. Tact yes. Subtlety none. Everyone is clear about where Violets stand in terms of their beliefs and values. Violets have clear internal moral codes that are evident in all they do and say.

> *"Managers do things right.
> Leaders do the right thing."*
> Warren Bennis

BORN ORATORS
Violets recognize the power of words and utilize them carefully and selectively; they appreciate seeing the effect their words have on others. They are clear about what they know and what they wish to convey to others.

Violets are the most natural orators and can speak effectively to large groups of people. Because they are also extremely private in their personal lives, not all Violets have experienced public speaking to know they can speak. Many are *so* private about their personal lives and feelings, that it stops them from stepping forward as teachers, leaders and orators.

Violets are very much at home when they speak and teach. It is a safe, comfortable space for them to share, even about themselves. In many ways, they are more intimate when they share with a crowd, even millions, than when they are asked to share one-on-one. This switch is confusing for others. For example, an observer, or a listener in the audience can be transformed by a Violet's speech; but when they approach them afterwards, expecting instant connection, they meet a very composed and unavailable person.

FEW CLOSE RELATIONSHIPS

Although they long for easy friendships, Violets avoid intimacy and closeness with most people because they feel they would overwhelm others. They also sense that many close relationships would scatter their personal power, and they are right. So Violets select their close relationships very carefully. The vastness of their minds and the charge of their energy fields would overwhelm many of us, if we got too close to them.

PASSIONATE INDIVIDUALS

The emotions of Violets can be larger than life. They struggle to accept the power in their rich emotional landscape; they only like this about themselves if there is a safe place or person to express it, someone that understands the grandness of their emotional energy, and allows them to express that energy with abandon.

Violets often have only one or two truly intimate relationships where they can be transparent, imperfect and passionate in this way. That one safe-harbor person is critical for them. As powerful as they are, they need that counterpart. Others will observe such relationships and see an imbalance of power, but they are mistaken. The counterpart person is more than justly rewarded for all the patience, space and service they provide their Violet partner, with depth, excitement, passion and tenderness. They have an exclusive role and feel it a privilege. Not everyone can be in that role, but Violets recognize their need and greatly value those who are willing and able to fill it.

For all the control they exude 95% of the time, Violets can be more reactionary and sensitive than any other personality the remaining 5% of the time. With all their passions, a temper simmers as well and, when it peaks, takes them and everyone else by surprise.

Because Violets often maintain a dominant position, it is shocking when you say something and see that you have really offended or hurt them. They often react in one of two ways: with anger and defensiveness, or with devastation and complete withdrawal. No matter how they react, it is always immediate, and it always feels like someone sucked all the air out of the room. The other person often does not know what happened.

The interesting thing with this reactive sensitivity in Violets is that whole families, corporations, and even governments can revolve around avoiding that kind of reaction from their Violet leader. They do not want to offend or hurt them, and they especially do not want to feel their wrath. The saying, "walking on eggshells," probably came from someone close to a Violet.

SELF-CRITICAL PERFECTIONISTS
Violets are extremely self-critical. They berate themselves and apologize for their weaknesses and the emotional things that they say. They learn to control their emotions at very young ages because they believe they are too much for others, and because they do not like anything to feel out-of-control. They are perfectionists in this way. There is no personality more private about their emotions and personal lives than Violets. For the most part, they need to remain this way in order to be able to provide all of the strength and vision they offer to the masses.

> *"I'm a perfectionist, so I can drive myself mad
> —and other people, too. At the same time,
> I think that's one of the reasons I'm successful.
> Because I really care about what I do."*
> Michelle Pfeiffer

CONTROL & SELF-MASTERY

They appear highly logical, which they are, but they are also highly emotional. They keep their emotions in check when they can, and put a lot of pressure on themselves to be composed. They can appear to be made of steel, are labeled "tough as nails," and others find them difficult to read and know because of their composure.

Violets set the bar for personal excellence, extending it to the rest of us by example. We hold them up as a standard of excellence and comparison because they are competent in so many things. They seem to communicate knowledge, mastery and control in all that they do. The rest of us admire and resent them for this perfectionistic composure.

EFFECTIVE SPEAKERS & TEACHERS

However composed they appear on the outside, Violets make decisions internally based on emotions and strong intuition, but they are generally able to present that information in a logical, practical fashion. Therein lies their power. This is a highly effective means of delivery because they are able to appeal to our intellect, our emotions and our spirit simultaneously.

Violets do not always recognize this effect and often think they are simply presenting a powerful logical position. Though their complexity and comprehensive understanding often remains under the surface, it is communicated to us loud and clear in all they say and do.

FEARLESSLY COMMITTED

Violets' self-mastery leads them to a sense of fearlessness and of their own personal power to bridle their passions and remain in control. The confidence they develop in their ability to take on the problems of life, their own and others, allows them to take on anything they choose and fully commit themselves, mind, body and soul.

> *"Circumstances do not make a man, they reveal him."*
> Wayne Dyer

CAPTAINS, MASTERS & SAVIORS

Violets are the captains of the ship, fearless and relentless in their ability to steer the individual or the masses to safety—whether those masses are a small group like a family, a larger group like a company, or on the grand scale, the world. They are single-minded in their leadership. The needy and destitute immediately feel a sense of protection and direction from Violets, and Violets often find themselves in parent or authority roles with others. They cannot help but rise to the occasion when others are struggling.

POWER TO CONSUME

The only thing Violets really need to watch is their tendency to overtake others who are weak, struggling, or young, in their efforts to protect or "save" them. Enveloping them in their own powerful energy field, Violets can end up making all of the decisions for others and fixing things for them instead of teaching independence. These codependent relationships can often happen between Violets and their children, employees, and friends-in-need.

CREATE DEPENDENCIES

Violets can choose friends simply based on how needy they are, rather than mutual need. It is important for Violets to be aware of this dynamic because, in trying to help others, they create dependency instead of self-sufficiency. The irony is that self-sufficiency is the natural state of Violets, so they are actually the best teachers of it. There are endless opportunities for Violets to pass this strength to others. They simply need to temper their encompassing power with some distance and objectivity, so the lesson comes through clearly.

DRIVEN TO LEAD & GUIDE

There is a balance between caretaking and leading for Violets to master. Violets truly need to show others the way. They have a very broad perspective of life and that is what they need to share with others, more than anything else. The more they become aware of this innate urging to lead and guide, the more careful and effective they become in changing lives for the better.

Control is what happens when they do not own this innate urging to lead. In all of our admiration of Violets, the thing that rubs us wrong is a sense that we are being controlled.

Regardless of the setting they are in, Violets have to lead and guide. Violets that do not have people to guide are like fish out of water—or tyrants without country. Some Violets lead quietly, others lead loudly, but lead they must.

Violets are "Masters of their Domain", and everyone within their reach knows it. At home, at work, at play or in politics Violets extend sphere-of-influence extends to the boundaries of all of these systems. Everyone and everything revolves around the law of the Violet and their particular value system. Anyone with Violet parents can attest to this: that their influence and power was far greater than that of anyone else in their whole world.

Violets eventually learn to own their power and how to wield it appropriately over time. But, it is a hard road for them. They find their immense capabilities difficult to digest and assimilate, and so they are hesitant to admit that the power is there. Interestingly, of all the personalities, Violets have the most difficulty accepting their Aura Personality.

Violet women are even more remiss in owning their power. This is primarily due to the social assumption that women should be passive and submissive. Violets are not bystanders in life; whatever their life is about, they engage in it completely. Violets are easy to identify by this trait, even if they are unwilling to own who they are.

> *"We still think of a powerful man as a born leader and a powerful woman as an anomaly."*
> Margaret Atwood

PARADOXICAL & INFLUENCING EITHER WAY

Violets are incredibly paradoxical in their behaviors. They can be: strict and flexible, righteous and unorthodox, public and private, perfectly controlled and spontaneously passionate. They tend to choose one extreme or another and whatever they choose is immediately impressed upon all around them. They are that influential.

For this reason, Violets are never really free to just live. The consequences of their choices always smack them in the face, reflected right back to them by those within their field-of-influence. Violets feel this burden and, can sometimes try to run from it, but they never really can.

VOCALIZING EXPERIENCE IS A RELEASE

To relieve some of the pressure of being a natural leader, Violets can verbally share what they are going through with those around them. They can also admit fault and apologize more. These gestures are not always easy for Violets, but they are incredibly liberating. Others gain from those actions as well; they gain perspective about the bumpiness of life and the infallibility of humans when they observe how Violets process inner turmoil. In this way, others, in turn, can become more forgiving in every aspect of their lives.

STANDARDS OF EXCELLENCE

For all their desire for personal privacy, Violets are on display as our standards of excellence; they may as well accept it instead of trying to will it otherwise.

> *We radiate who we are all of the time,*
> *whether we like it or not.*
> *So we may as well own ourselves*
> *and stand in our power.*

It is always interesting to meet Violets who have not consciously stepped into their power—they actually believe they have succeeded in concealing their immense energy field just by using controlled voices and composed statures. Violets control many things in their lives, so it is a bit of a surprise to them to realize they haven't been hiding their power from anyone. On the flip side, Violets who own their power are like national monuments; moral beacons to all they encounter, especially those within the reach of their voices.

CRITICAL BECAUSE ALL IS VISIBLE TO THEM
Violets are so aware of everything that it is hard for them to hold back criticism of themselves and others. If their mission to lead, guide, teach and influence is misdirected or thwarted, they can become critical and controlling of their immediate surroundings, including the people within their vicinity. They channel their forceful energy into containers not nearly big enough to hold it. It feels really controlling to those around them because Violets are so powerful. Violets do not see their power as clearly as others do. They just feel compelled to extend it. They are constantly reaching for equilibrium within themselves and a space big enough to hold all that they are.

EGO BATTLE
In order to channel and use their powerful energy comfortably, effectively and appropriately, there is one significant and interesting transformation necessary: this happens when Violets willingly surrender their Ego. The way to surrender Ego is by facing their power, owning it, and then recognizing from whence it comes: from God.

> *"Learning how to be still,*
> *to really be still and let life happen—*
> *that stillness becomes a radiance."*
> Morgan Freeman

If Violets choose not to surrender Ego, they can spend their lives ping-ponging between anxiety and anger. These miserable Violets are like forest fires, inevitably engulfing others with their misery. Their misdirected energy eventually dissipates just as a fire burns itself out. This is because Ego power is not that effective in the long run. That said, Violets who have surrendered to and partnered with their all-powerful God, on the other hand, are stunning. They are stunning eternal flames whose effects are endlessly rippling outward.

> *"Man is immortal, not because he alone among creatures has an inexhaustible voice, but because he has a soul, a spirit capable of compassion and sacrifice and endurance."*
> Morgan Freeman

VIOLET FAMOUS PEOPLE*
George Washington—former U.S. president
Martin Luther King, Jr.—civil rights leader
Winston Churchill—British Prime Minister, orator & historian
David Hawkins (Indigo)—psychiatrist, author & teacher
Leo Tolstoy—writer
Morgan Freeman—actor
Ben Kingsley—actor
Tom Cruise—actor
Judi Dench—actor
Julie Andrews—actor
Michelle Pfeiffer (Green-Amber)—actor
Denzel Washington (Blue-Amber)—actor
Robert Duvall—actor
Maggie Smith (Blue-Amber)—actor
Wayne Dyer (Yellow)—thought leader, speaker & author

Aslan

Sauron

*Parentheses signify the secondary part of their main Aura Personality.

~

THE LAVENDER AURA PERSONALITY

The Free Spirit

"We live in fact in a world starved for solitude, silence, and private: and therefore starved for meditation and true friendship."
From *The Weight of Glory, and Other Addresses*,
By C.S. Lewis

FREE SPIRITS

Lavenders are reminiscent of all winged creatures, real and mythical—angels, faeries, birds and butterflies—likewise lovely, elusive and given to flight. And, like exotic butterflies, if one gently lands upon your shoulder, stay quiet and still; it just might linger with you for a while.

These creative, gentle souls touch lightly upon the earth and other people. Any time you spend with Lavenders is their gift to you. Be grateful when you get it, never demand it, and they just might keep giving it.

SENSITIVE

Lavenders are tenderhearted, emotionally in-tune, accepting people. They are generally very easy to be around, but when they are down, they tend to brood like Blues and Violets. They also hold grudges and do not forgive easily. Because they spend a lot of energy trying to please others, it is very difficult for them to assimilate unkindness from others.

Lavenders are obvious when they are upset, though they like to think they are keeping it from others with silence and hiding out. They are not fooling anyone; their behavior when upset is so drastically different from how they are when they are happy and at peace with the world. Where Blues openly pout, Lavenders do so in silence. But, that does not make it any less apparent to those that are close to them.

AMAZING FRIENDS

Overall, Lavenders are very likeable people and, although they do not ask for it, others tend to cluster around them. They enjoy people and prefer undemanding, casual settings for interacting with others.

QUIETLY HUMOROUS

Lavenders have a great sense of humor. They can be both silly and witty, but are generally quiet about it. Only those in close proximity catch their clever commentary. Lavenders are not humorous for attention, but for enjoyment. They have naturally good boundaries with humor, knowing instinctively how much to say and when to say it. Lavenders are innately tactful, never overdone.

SOCIAL INTELLIGENCE
People watch Lavenders for social cues in a variety of settings. Lavenders clearly understand and incorporate social rules but, instead of raising themselves above others for it, they tend to be generous and gracious with those who fumble socially. Lavenders add grace to others and find awkward people endearing. They are unselfish with their compliments and with their friendship, especially with those who truly need it.

NONJUDGMENTAL
Lavenders are not judgmental, and they are naturally accepting of everyone and everything. They are perfectly fine being in the background in most situations. They usually occupy the less dominant role in all of their relationships—be it friendship, parent-child, or romance. For all of these reasons, Lavenders appear to be ideal companions, especially for the more dominant Aura Personalities. And, if they are not being controlled or manipulated by their partners, they can be ideal companions.

OFTEN KEEP TO RELATIONSHIP SIDELINES
The fragile and delicate side of Lavenders brings out the protective instincts in others, while their elusiveness can bring out a questing instinct, making them targets for romantic masochists. In their minds, Lavenders believe they are actively looking for love, but in reality they never feel quite ready for it to arrive. Lavenders often find themselves in these *almost* relationships that never quite materialize; it is easier for them to daydream about

romance than actually have it. The very nature of romantic relationships-a constant expectation for interaction-impedes on the privacy and solitude Lavenders require.

In any kind of relationship with Lavenders, the thing to understand is that they need their freedom. Like all winged creatures, Lavenders must be able to sense that, at any time, they can leave: leave the room, leave the party, leave the conversation, or even leave the country, if need be. If Lavenders know freedom and privacy are available, then they are safe to stay. Lavenders desire attachment to others. Their gauge for safety and freedom is just fine-tuned and specific—it requires an escape pod. So if others respect this, they will have great relationships with Lavenders.

This does not mean Lavenders cannot have committed relationships or children and families of their own. It simply means they must have room for their expansive natures alongside their relationships.

Lavenders need to roam and experience the landscapes, textures and peoples they create in their minds, as well as those they encounter through travel. In a nutshell, Lavenders must always provide two things for themselves: (1) Alone time to daydream without expectation or pressure from others, and (2) Vacations, other experiences, or other forms of travel where they explore new places, ideas and cultures.

PROLIFIC DAYDREAMERS
One of the strongest gifts of Lavenders is their ability to daydream. No one else matches them in exploring the world of imagination. Observing from the outside, it is

as if they literally inhabit two realms, and not simultaneously; one is the realm of reality where the rest of us hang out; the other is the realm of imagination.

CREATIVELY FERTILE IMAGINATIONS

To call Lavenders creative is a gross understatement—worlds without end are manifest in their imaginings. Often they are not even aware of the extent of their creative abilities because so much of it remains in the form of thought. In fact, very little of what they imagine makes it out of their minds. Lavenders have low external output but are internally hyper-productive. We might only see the tip of the iceberg in their organized creative offerings, but their creativity colors everything they touch all throughout their lives.

Very different from Magentas who are in a constant state of impulsive creation, Lavenders need much stillness and alone time, compared to what they manifest in the material realm. Alone time is any time where freeform mind meanderings can occur, which include, among other things, naps, taking walks, sitting in the sun, watching films, or doing a mundane activity with their hands. Lavenders are even creative in how they find time to be alone with their imaginations. They are unaware that they do this because it is synonymous with breathing for them.

> *"Our imagination flies—*
> *we are its shadow on the earth."*
> Vladimir Nabokov

Lavenders have mastered the art of being alone in a room full of people. They can even check out in the middle of conversations without others noticing, responding on cue while simultaneously engaging in their own imaginations. When you call them out for their half-attention, they always laugh. They are well aware of what they have been getting away with in conversations, knowing that most people have no idea.

DAYDREAMING IS THEIR PRODUCTIVITY

Viewing daydreaming as a gift to be encouraged and cultivated is a new way of thinking for most people. Lavenders usually count it a curse in themselves. But think of life without the starkly beautiful, universal truths given to us from those seemingly futile ruminations in Lavender minds. Lavenders are the truly, poignantly artistic souls. All the labels we attach to artists apply most directly to Lavenders: creative, perfectionists, noncommittal, self-doubting, self-critical, nonconformists and impractical.

> *"I think I could learn*
> *a little patience with myself*
> *if I took a view of myself that included*
> *concepts like dormancy (instead of laziness),*
> *seed planting (instead of just scattered),*
> *gestation (instead of doing-something-right-this-second)."*
> From *Prayers from a NonBeliever*, Julia Cameron

PERFECTIONISTS

Whether writing novels, poems, painting, designing, or creating any other art form, Lavenders are perfectionists, critical of their creations and unnecessarily critical of their low production. They judge themselves against social standards for productivity. They often do not call themselves artists because they cannot quite picture doing art full-time, nor can they imagine getting paid for their fertile imaginations. But pay we would if we could get a tiny glimpse of their minds.

NATURALLY GIVING

Lavenders give many treasures of infinite value to us, along with their creations, namely; friendship, peace, kindness, unique individuality, a sense of inclusion, and permission to live more freely, creatively, and easily in this world. It is a blessing to have Lavenders in your life. They are like personalized angels that flit in and out at whim. Bringing with them complete acceptance and a sense of wonder for the rare experience it is to share in a really special friendship.

Although they cannot see this in themselves, Lavenders are treasures. They are amazingly sympathetic and compassionate listeners that do not feel the need to advise or judge. That is part of what makes them such amazing friends. So rather than ask more of them, appreciate what they give, and you will have true friends for life.

Because of their need for alone time, Lavenders approach all relationships tentatively. They appear to be loners because they always maintain a bit of emotional distance in relationships. This distance actually gives them room to flourish and makes them capable of caring for others, while simultaneously preserving their sense of safety. Nonetheless, Lavenders feel other's need to be closer and more committed and they judge themselves as inadequate in relationships because of it. This dynamic is painful for them because they care deeply for others and do not like to create disappointment.

GIVE OF THEMSELVES & THEN WITHDRAW

Lavenders have the gift of love for others akin to Blues. The difference is how deep they go into relationship waters. Blues jump into intimacy with both feet and are fulfilled and nourished in the intensity. Lavenders tend to dip their toes, maybe get their feet wet, only to find themselves often stepping right back out of emotional waters.

The other difference between Blues and Lavenders is that Lavenders care so much they cannot stop giving. As a natural consequence, they lose themselves and then flee the relationship in an effort to regain their sense of self. This pattern is not the only way, but it is often what Lavenders do until they learn appropriate emotional boundaries in relationships.

CODEPENDENCY & ROMANTICISM
Blues and Lavenders have other relationship and life lessons in common. They are both romantics with tendencies toward codependency and pedestalling others, always to be let down. Like Blues, Lavenders are also disappointed by reality because it is such a far cry from the people and places of their imaginations.

Lavenders have less of a barrier around their energy fields than Blues. They are periodically flooded by the energy of others, but they also tend to seek out stimulation, whereas Crystals tend to avoid it.

TRAVELLERS
In particular, Lavenders love the stimulation of newness—new places, new cultures, and new people. They love every part of the process of getting to know something new, and nothing provides as many sources of "new" like travel. Lavenders step off the train or plane and are immediately in their natural element; what they often experience in their imaginings is suddenly rolled out before them in reality.

Travel is the yellow brick road, red carpet, and magic carpet ride for Lavenders. The sights, smells, faces, energy, food, and tradition; the intimacy in meeting the eyes of strangers, of children; the opportunities for spontaneity; all of these things are fuel for their expansive souls. Youth hostels, humanitarian volunteer groups, study abroad programs, and spiritual pilgrimages all over the globe are filled with Lavenders. Collectively, they are exploring the world, finding the nook-and-cranny villages in the remotest locations.

INSTANT LOVE FOR STRANGERS

Travel also provides another crucial experience that Lavenders do not usually find in other ways—an opportunity to love immediately and unconditionally. Lavenders have a unique ability to love strangers instantly. Strangers become family in a short time. Lavenders love easily and their hearts soften quickly when they feel that someone is in greater need of love. For some reason, with strangers, Lavenders feel that need and give that kind of love without reservation.

In these days, weeks or even months of travel, Lavenders fall in love with entire cultures, and the people within those cultures. As a result, Lavenders feel a sense of accomplishment and a satisfaction in their souls that is rarely felt otherwise. Giving of themselves fully, and getting their need for creative stimulation met simultaneously, Lavenders expand.

Contrary to what they believe, Lavenders do not have to travel to achieve this state of unity within. They can find it wherever they are, or bring it with them wherever they go. Meeting strangers with a different background from their own and exposure to new things will allow them to be their expansive selves. They can seek out the unique and avant-garde that surrounds us wherever we are if we look for them.

FUTURE-ORIENTED

Because Lavenders are in the creative process in their minds most of the time, they are forward-thinkers—future-oriented. This is fine and necessary for their creativity, but it can also mean they often miss the wonders of the present. Learning to be present helps Lavenders find great satisfaction wherever they are. This also helps them value the people in their current relationships. Lavenders can have a bit of an addiction to leaving the old for the new, even when that is not what they really want or need. By choosing to consciously engage in the present, they allow for the newness they crave and provide a sense of belonging.

Lavenders can expand and share their gifts of love and creation wherever they are. They just need time alone and change to serve as fuel for their giving. Life stays fresh if change is plentiful.

BORN UNIQUE

As small children, Lavenders love pretend play and their imaginations are more outwardly apparent. As they age, they play with fashion and social trends. They find clothing and fashion to be great outlets for their creativity. Fashion is a way to set themselves apart as unique and nonconforming. Lavenders are fashion setters for the rest of us because they are always one step ahead and adding their own twist to whatever is currently trendy. None of their creative play is for attention, but they cannot help wanting to be acknowledged for their uniqueness. Lavenders recognize that their internal world is very different from the one played out in front of them by the rest of us, and they need us to know that.

EXPERIMENTAL
Lavenders can be very experimental because they are naturally open to ideas and people, especially unorthodox ones. This is a great trait, but can get them into trouble since Lavenders do not always have clarity about what is safe, or good for them, and what is not.

Lavenders are often quiet about their explorations and interests. Sometimes the only way you know anything about what is going on is by the clothes they wear and the music they listen to. During teenage years and into early adulthood, Lavenders try on different hats instead of just wearing their own. They are aware early on that their thoughts and ideas are not mainstream, and they have a difficult time being true to themselves. They vacillate between being true to themselves and trying to please others.

COMPLIANT & REBELLIOUS
As they are exploring identity, Lavenders can go through a period of quiet rebellion (or not so quiet, for their parents and siblings, at least). They do not respond positively to rules, boundaries or feeling controlled; unless they intuitively know the imposer has good intentions. Lavenders would rather not rock the boat, so if authority figures have good intentions, Lavenders will comply and even help.

Lavenders tend to vacillate between pleasing others and complying, and isolating from others and being hyper-independent. Living with them is a push-pull experience.

It can be difficult to know where you really stand in relationship to them.

Lavenders are free spirits that naturally long for freedom from social constraints and traditional expectations. They have no need to impose their uniqueness on others, or to rebel, but they need the choice to opt in or out available to them at all times.

IMPRESSIONABLE & NEED BOUNDARIES

For all of their open-mindedness and openness to exploration, Lavenders are very impressionable. They need to choose carefully what they expose themselves to. They are not naturally careful about this but they eventually learn to be, with experience. Their imaginations and actual adventures can take them much further than the rest of us could ever conceive; they might find themselves, one too many times, in situations they would rather not be in. Lavenders have to learn their own boundaries and honor them in order to expand safely into who they are.

> *"Fear is an insidious and deadly thing.*
> *It can warp judgment, freeze reflexes,*
> *and breed mistakes.*
> *Worse, it's contagious."*
> Jimmy Stewart

INTUITIVELY AWARE OF POSSIBILITIES

Being halfway in imagination and halfway in reality provides Lavenders with a unique angle on life. The realm of what is possible is so much greater in their minds. In many ways Lavenders literally see, hear and feel more than the rest of us with what is generally referred to as ESP (extra-sensory perception) abilities. They spend more time in the eyes-half shut theta state than the rest of us, where lines between reality and alternate realities wear thin. They have obvious intuitive gifts in this regard.

NATURALLY PSYCHIC

Many of us are aware that there is much more to our existence than what is physically manifest, but Lavenders' eyes are actually open to those larger realms from very early ages. Like the rest of us, they may be told to see what is acceptable and "not see" what is not, because that is how we are socialized, but many Lavenders are able to hold onto their "sixth" sense. All Lavenders are sensitive to "other-worldly" things, but only some choose to develop and consciously use those abilities.

Lavenders with a heightened sixth sense have the gift of intuition. They can seem overly sensitive to others and, in fact, they are, but their gifts lie within that sensitivity, acuity and awareness.

> *"Life is a spiritual dance*
> *and our unseen partner has steps to teach us*
> *if we will allow ourselves to be led.*
> *The next time you are restless,*
> *remind yourself it is the universe asking*
> *'Shall we dance?'"*
> Julia Cameron

Those with high intuition instinctively gather volumes of information about that which is not readily seen, heard or felt by the rest of us, and there are a variety of ways they use this information. Some Lavenders feel burdened by their abilities, while others see them as opportunities to learn and grow. The interesting choice for Lavenders is not to decide whether or not they are psychic, because they are; the truly interesting choice is whether or not they are going to become conscious, responsible, and conscientious for their intuitive abilities.

NEED FOR BOUNDARIES AROUND GIFTS
There is a great need for Lavenders to create boundaries around their gifts and how they are used. By doing so, those gifts become a blessing in their lives and the lives of others, instead of a burden or a drain. Lavenders are easily lost in the lives of others, as well as in all that is otherworldly. The way to find themselves is to consciously live in the present, maintaining their own life as their first and truest obligation.

LAVENDER FAMOUS PEOPLE*
Walt Disney—Imagineer extraordinaire
Jimmy Stewart (Blue-Amber)—actor
C.S. Lewis (Amber)—author & thought leader
Dr. Seuss-author & artist
Julia Cameron—author & teacher
Tori Amos—singer & songwriter
Stephanie Meyer (Green)—author
Jennifer Love-Hewitt (Green-Amber)—actor & producer
Scarlett Johansson—actor

*Parentheses signify the secondary part of their main Aura Personality.

THE SPIRITUAL FAMILY

~

AURA PERSONALITIES

The Spiritual Aura Personalities

The Spiritual Aura Personalities are energy people. They operate from the vibrations they feel. This is a different experience from loud bodily sensations or lucid thoughts. They are primarily taking information through intuition and inspiration, with their radars tuned into universal messages of light and dark, truth and falsehood, expansion and contraction.

The Spiritual Aura Personalities feel like sojourners rather than permanent residents here on earth. If they do not stay close to God, the darkness easily consumes them. If they do, then they are at peace in their sojourn, ready to lead the rest of us into light with their lives of integrity.

The Spiritual Aura Personalities are:

CRYSTALS
INDIGOS
AVENTURINE-CRYSTALS
MAGENTA-CRYSTALS
AMETHYST-CRYSTALS
INDIGO-CRYSTALS
IMPERIAL TOPAZES

~

THE CRYSTAL AURA PERSONALITY

The Vessel

"[Galadriel] held up a small crystal phial: it glittered as she moved it, and rays of white light sprang from her hand. "In this phial," she said, "is caught the light of Eärendil's star, set amid the waters of my fountain. It will shine still brighter when night is about you. May it be a light to you in dark places, when all other lights go out."
From *The Fellowship of The Ring*, by J.R.R. Tolkien

CONTAINERS OF LIGHT
Crystals are vessels of light, yet they are oblivious to that fact, and to the effect their brightness has on others. Crystals are vessels or containers for many things,

including the energy of other people. This is their great gift and their Achilles heel until they master what they let in. The trick for Crystals is to let the light within them shine so purely that there is no way for any darkness to enter. This is a lifelong lesson for Crystals that teaches them many eternal concepts and principles.

> *"Today you overwhelm my most lovingness*
> *by how strangely deep you go*
> *into, through, and around me."*
> From the poem, *Prayer of Being*, by Alan Harris

GIFT OF FAITH

Crystal energy embodies an enduring faith in God and His eternal purposes. Crystals are faithful because so much of what they do and how they serve is hidden from them, as are the purposes behind their trials and shortcomings. Despite their blindness, Crystals go forward in faith.

> *"Blessed are the pure in heart:*
> *for they shall see God."*
> *The Holy Bible*, Matthew 5:8

CHILDLIKE & NAIVE

Crystals are playful, joyful, pure-in-heart souls that bring healing with them wherever they go. They have the gentle, sensitive, impressionable nature of children but, unlike other children growing into adulthood, Crystals retain these childlike qualities all throughout their lives. This is part of the reason they seem, and even look, younger than their age. In so many ways Crystals feel very young and more like children than adults, even well into adulthood. This is especially true when it comes to making decisions for themselves. Crystals have to learn to accept responsibility in order to fully transition into adulthood.

Crystals are late bloomers in many ways, including how they handle emotional disappointments and upsets. They have a tendency to react like children when they feel helpless. Crystals get stuck in emotions and cannot see their way out. They sometimes throw tantrums and lash out at those around them. They have difficulty looking at the big picture, or even acknowledging all of the immediate details when they feel hurt. To them, there are many realities in life too stark to look at directly. By trying to protect themselves by not facing things however, Crystals end up stuck in the experience and cannot move into a place where they can get a clear perspective or an appropriate context. Their fear, more often than not, creates more of what they are afraid of.

On the flip side, Crystals manifest the virtues of childlike behavior along with their childish overreactions. Crystals are vulnerable, teachable, humble, spontaneous and trusting. They laugh easily, forgive quickly and love everyone. Crystals are open to everything good. The have an instant desire for things to be made right and for peace and harmony to descend upon all situations, if possible.

DECISION PARALYSIS
Crystals never feel adequately equipped, or mature enough to make decisions. They would prefer a more confident and, in their eyes, more competent person to make all of their decisions for them. Crystals are constantly asking others to provide information and guidance for their lives. Many difficulties they experience in life are in direct correlation to their constant state of

perplexity. In fact, Crystals can be indecisive, to the point of paralysis, in moving forward in their lives.

SELF-DOUBT IS THEIR NEMESIS
Crystals are filled with self-doubt about all that they think, say and do; they do not trust their ability to make correct choices for themselves or for others. This constant second-guessing looks like procrastination and laziness on the outside but, on the inside, great turmoil is raging. Inner battles are being fought that, if not won, they believe might ruin everything.

Another piece to their puzzling dispositions is that Crystals always want to do what is right. This is an interesting desire since they struggle trusting themselves enough to ever know what "right" is.

Crystals feel like they somehow missed some essential instructions and information that everyone else instinctively knows. This constant state of "not knowing," and trying to figure things out places them in a state of anxiety and victimhood but, it also creates an openness to learning new information, and new ways of doing things, unmatched by any other personality.

A MIRROR FOR OTHERS
Crystals are like mirrors, portals, or conduits for inspiration and light to travel through. They are empaths who feel hopeless, lost and unknown even to themselves. Because their gifts are so specific and uncommon, they rarely see them exemplified by others and are rarely able to identify them in themselves.

PUT OTHERS AT EASE
One thing Crystals notice, even at young ages in their lives, is that others feel an immediate ease around them.

Without understanding why, others feel safe and understood around Crystals. And it goes one step further than feeling understood. Around Crystals, others suddenly understand themselves. They see themselves much more clearly than they did before, like a mirror of their soul has been held up before them. In the same way crystal quartz responds to light, Crystals unknowingly amplify the personality traits of others with their reflective listening and presence. They are like prisms, absorbing, fracturing and dispersing the rainbow light of the other Aura Personalities.

> *"I think it's impossible to really know someone,*
> *what they want, what they believe,*
> *and not love them the way they love themselves."*
> From *Enders Game*, by Orson Scott Card

EMPATHY OR IDENTITY CONFUSION

Crystals have the ability to consider the experiences of a multitude of people at the same time. As a consequence, they spend a lot of time accommodating people. With their ability to know first-hand what others experience energetically, Crystals can go a step beyond being pleasers and into the realm of codependency, if they are not watchful.

Information about others registers within Crystals' own energetic systems. In psychology this ability is termed over-identification. In reality, it is a gift called empathy that, when used correctly, can benefit everyone involved. Learning how to use it correctly, however, takes a bit of time and practice.

Crystals are empaths, but they do not usually know it because what others perceive as empathy, Crystals unfortunately experience as identity confusion. Crystals feel like whomever they are with, and as a consequence, have difficulty distinguishing their own feelings from the feelings of others. In this struggle, empathy is present, and though others benefit from it, Crystals are in the dark about it. Ironically, Crystal empaths—those who can immediately and completely experience the energy of others—are blind to their own energy and its attending gifts.

The best way for Crystals to find out who they are is to experience themselves through other people, and to learn to distinguish the other Aura Personalities from their own. For Crystals, discovering Aura Personalities as a classification system is like blind people discovering Braille. For the first time the world opens up wide enough for them to get a glimpse of their abilities and, with this knowledge, they realize they will never be in darkness again.

ABSORB & INTERNALIZE EVERYTHING
Being blind to their gifts, and unable to instinctively separate themselves from others, creates a weak emotional and psychic barrier for Crystals. Everything, in turn, feels personal to Crystals—like they are targets and things are happening to them that they are unable to stop. They can actually go through the whole range of body and psychic responses to tragedy, even if they are just witnessing, reading, or hearing about it, especially when they are unaware of their openness.

Often when Crystals witness violence of any kind in their environment, or even in the media, they exhibit the same complex symptoms of post-traumatic stress disorder as abuse victims. To put it mildly, Crystals internalize everything.

Like no others, Crystals can experience extreme fatigue during or after a busy, high-energy outing—like a concert, party or large gathering of any kind. Add anything extra to the mix and the need to purge the energy afterwards will be even greater. Things that can be over-stimulating for Crystals include: music, loud noises, lots of people, multiple conversations happening at once, any kind of spectacle to watch, darkness, or even lots of lights.

HYPER PLUGGED-IN TO THE ENVIRONMENT
During such events, Crystals match the energy around them. They seem to be the person most engaged or "plugged in" to their environment. They are so present wherever they are that Crystals become the easiest power source for every energy circuit to plug into for grounding. This is why Crystals become chameleons to their environment. They are taking on the energy of everything around them. They ride the environmental current, and afterward they inevitably crash.

WEIGHTED BY ENERGY OF OTHERS
Like a sponge, they soak up much more sensory input than any other personality. They get heavily weighed down and, like an overloaded hard drive on a computer, they become useless with all the conflicting and unfamiliar input and data.

RESPONSIBLE FOR THEIR ENVIRONMENT
The first step for Crystals in wringing out or energetically detoxing from negativity is to become conscious of it. The next step involves releasing the energy with words or activities. This step usually involves talking it out in a step-by-step, play-by-play fashion, the way psychological

aftereffects of any trauma are handled. This is often the fastest way for healing to happen for Crystals. Purging through talking can be taxing on those listening, unless they know the purpose and remain separate. Lastly, Crystals need to incorporate peaceful rituals into their daily lives as a counterbalance to negativity and darkness. Peaceful rituals might include things like: spending time in solitude or nature, praying, meditating, doing conscious breath work, drinking water, practicing Yoga or T'ai chi ch'uan, sleeping, writing, or making art.

Crystals are truly sensitive creatures and need to learn how to protect their energy fields. If they choose not to, they will remain in a state of hopeless victimhood, powerless to access their gifts and grab ahold of their lives. If they choose to learn, their gifts can help heal and wring out the negativity of the entire planet.

NATURAL HEALERS

Being so automatically plugged in to the energy fields of everything around them, Crystals make the most natural healers. They perceive so easily the pain and discord within others and easily access healing energy from all kinds of positive sources. Much of the healing work that happens through Crystals is unconscious. Crystals are unaware of the healing energy they access, but they do sense when others are experiencing wholeness.

SPIRITUAL CONDUITS

A major role of Crystals is to serve as conduits for heavenly things. It is their natural inclination and part of the reason for their profound desire to think and do things that are "right" and without guile. If they are in rightness, or have pure intentions, they are able to connect others to the universal healing and "rightness" available to all of us.

SUSCEPTIBLE TO FEAR
Another difficult task for them is to come to terms with the harshness of the world. To gain added perspective and accept the darker side of life, including illness, tragedy, violence, and evil, they must learn not to fear these things. That does not mean Crystals need to embrace dark things in their lives. They need to recognize that judgment and fear block their ability to heal and teach. If Crystals can learn that everything serves God's purposes, that everything is for our growth and joy, and that the Plan is perfectly and mercifully created, then they can blossom and radiate their empathic love the way they were designed to.

SUFFERING IS THEIR TEACHER
A further challenge for Crystals is their overly sensitive physiological systems and weak immune systems. Crystals can spend a lot of time in physical illness or discord, from infancy onward and, if they are not careful, it is another way for them to justify a sense of victimhood.

SPIRITUAL GUIDES
The truth of their sensitive systems is that their bodies are their greatest teachers. Crystals experience ongoing pain with its accordant symptoms of psychological, emotional and spiritual suffering. As a result, they become empathic and compassionate healers. At the same time, traveling the plains of fear and powerlessness that so often accompany chronic pain and illness, Crystals have another opportunity to become spiritual guides for others. If they choose, with God, they can

transform that fear and powerlessness into something whole and powerful that encompasses faith, love and peaceful, personal power.

Crystals are sparkly no matter what, but when they overcome fear and give love permission to dominate their experience, they are beings of pure brilliant, shimmering peace and light. Crystals are a gift from God to those who honor their purity of intention.

CRYSTAL FAMOUS PEOPLE*
Mohandas Gandhi (Amber)—peaceful liberator
J.R.R. Tolkien—author
Chris Martin—lead singer, songwriter & pianist
Hrithik Roshan (Green-Amber)—actor
Natalie Portman (Indigo)—actor
Leonardo DiCaprio (Indigo)—actor

*Parentheses signify the secondary part of their main Aura Personality.

~

AURA PERSONALITIES

THE INDIGO
AURA PERSONALITY

The Paradigm-Shifter

"The most important persuasion tool you have in your entire arsenal is integrity."
Zig Ziglar

TRUE TO THEMSELVES
Indigos are what the rest of us seek in ourselves—they are true to themselves, no matter what. This constant mandate to be true to self is impossible for them to disobey—an obedience that is very attractive and refreshing to the rest of us. Fully actualized Indigos, manifest on the outside, the truth they know on the inside. The rest of us fall short striving toward such

internal and external harmony, so we look to Indigos to show us the way. They become the new standard to live by.

CONNECTED TO NATURE'S RHYTHMS

Indigos have a new kind of energy, one that runs in harmony with the energies of the earth. They are tracking so much energetically, in fact, that they are only capable of one outward task at a time. The pace of others is absurd to Indigos. Their pace is slower, connected to natural rhythms. Their hearts are strong and constant, and it feels good and peaceful to join their pace.

Indigos are tapped into currents of the earth, the ocean, and gravity, sound; as well as, animals, people, societies, and prevailing thought forms. Everything is vibrating and Indigos are catching each wave. They are in rhythm with the electromagnetic realm and resonate with it. This connection is void of emotion; it is energetic and vibrational. That is why Indigos can seem so antisocial and detached. They are just having a totally unique experience on this earth that most others cannot relate to.

Running purely on instinct, Indigos feel a constant, unsettling rush to lay down energetic cable lines for those who follow—specifically the New Crystals. Indigos have been and still are prepping humanity for the special vibrations New Crystals bring.

TECHNOLOGY IS ONE OF THEIR LANGUAGES

Technology was born and developed into young adulthood, at hyper-speed, through Indigos because they understand its rhythm. Technology is a first language for them; so are math, engineering, art and, especially, music. Indigo brains resonate far more naturally and harmoniously with these things than they do with people.

> *"By giving people the power to share,
> we're making the world more transparent."*
> Mark Zuckerberg

VIBRATIONALLY ATTUNED

Their attunement with all vibrations is not something they learn, it is something they are. In fact, the rest of us are seeking attunement with Indigo minds. It's why they are arrogant and why they are know-it-alls. They are literally experiencing the world more holistically than anyone else. They feel the interconnectedness of everything and, when we are quiet, the rest of us feel their harmonious vibration.

Indigos tend to join fully with one rhythm or another— whether through computers and technology, or by living close to nature, with their animals. They are rarely in mainstream careers or lifestyles and, if they are, they connect with the more natural rhythms energetically during their time off from work.

> *"Look deep into nature,
> and then you will understand
> everything better."*
> Albert Einstein

HIDE THEIR WISDOM

For the first part of their lives, Indigos feel unseen and unsure. They don't know how to share their truth and all they know from an energetic level. They learn right away that they do not want to lose their connection to natural rhythms because it feels so much better than society's harried pace. Indigos go into hiding to protect themselves, figuratively speaking. But they still follow their own directives, secretly riding the rhythms all the while.

ENERGETICALLY INSTINCTIVE
Indigos hide by hyper-focusing on things like simulation and strategy games and all types of technology. They go into fantasy realms where they can hone in on and run on their energetic instincts. They can literally hide even in a room full of people. Others often forget they are there. Indigos have the ability to stay off radar and energetically fade into the background. This is a self-preservation technique that allows them to hold onto what is true and real for them internally, while still observing and learning about things externally—like social customs.

These techniques are useful for a while, but eventually an awakening or accounting has to take place for Indigos where they begin to shift their internal lives into the external realm. Sometimes all it takes is one person acknowledging that they are not living true, or saying, "I know about you and who you really are." When Indigos are recognized, it is like they take a sudden inhale of breath for the first time since they decided to shut down as children. A few sensitive adults will be aware of Indigos when they are very young but for most, the awakening happens during their teenage or young adult years.

MAGNETIC
Despite their efforts to hide, people are still aware of and drawn to these unique, internally driven individuals. Indigos, however, are not usually aware of the magnetic

effect they have on others. In fact, because social rules are the one area of life that completely elude them, Indigos often do not trust the motives of others, and are wary when others are drawn to them. Indigos live in a paradox of not caring what others think and, simultaneously, striving to fit in socially.

SOCIALLY CLUELESS
The social experience for Indigos is that they are excluded; somehow missing out on the joke that everyone else is in on. They can be terribly insecure in relationships, often too serious and fairly unreadable. This is perplexing and frustrating for all involved because Indigos truly want, need and enjoy human connections.

Indigos need at least one person with whom they are truly intimate, and they need that intimacy to go both ways—the other person has to be willing to be completely open and vulnerable with them as well. Indigos can become possessive of their loved ones. They can become too fearful of losing them and, consequently, hold on too tightly.

ADMIRE PEOPLE TRUE TO THEMSELVES
They struggle with feelings of isolation and awkwardness, aware that they "stand out" and are somehow apart from others. They do not like this distinction and would love to feel at ease around others like Yellows, Reds, and a few others. Those they admire are not all socially inclined, but they are all comfortable with others and do not try to be what they are not. They recognize their place in the social order of things. Indigos have a blind spot in this way.

From birth, Indigos are searching for a place to offer their depth, seriousness and wisdom. Since they rarely come across those who understand them, they often dismiss this, shrugging off the deeper traits of their soul in exchange for feeling normal and mainstream.

But, alas, there is nothing mainstream about Indigos. For one, they are more energetically connected with others than the rest of us and will often drop close connection with all but one or two people. They have a great need to disconnect and remain separate and aloof. They cannot stay connected to natural rhythms if they tune in too closely to people and their constant disharmony.

INTENSELY AWARE
Though we often think of Indigos as cold and unfeeling, one moment of eye contact with them is enough to teach us that there is much emotional depth in them just beneath the surface. Eye contact with Indigos is like a warm embrace, a sudden intense awareness that someone has truly seen your soul and, in that moment, you tune into the deeper, natural rhythms they inhabit. Indigos sense this profound effect they have on others at early ages and learn to be cautious and selective about connecting, unsure of what to do with the responsibility.

INBORN SELF-CONFIDENCE
Many of us mistake the social awkwardness of Indigos as low self-esteem, but do not be fooled. No one is more innately self-confident than Indigos. There is nothing anyone can do to take that sense of self away. Indigos cannot be broken. They can be off base, but not broken.

> *"Insecurities are about as useful as trying to put the pin back in the grenade."*
> Brandon Boyd

Indigos' senses of self, and their self-directedness, are inborn, with no connection to outside directives or expectations (much to the chagrin of those who have stewardship over them). It can rankle them that they struggle socially, because they do not really struggle in any other way.

CREATE THEIR OWN LIFE CURRICULUM

Indigos accept their directives; they are who they are. That is how they live all of the time. If they decide to learn something that is in alignment with what they know of themselves, they easily embody it in every way. Indigos choose what they learn and when they learn it. They can succeed at anything, if they decide to. Whatever they decide to do, they become it inside and out, around and through, but others can often be left to deal with the fallout.

HIGHEST RESPONSIBILITY IS TO SELF

Indigos are lone rangers that do not assume responsibility for the lives of others—even those whose lives are intimately connected to their own. It must be a choice they make. They simply march forward to their own mandates, accepting the consequences of their chosen path, and deflecting everything that falls outside of their realm of responsibility.

CRITICAL & UNTRUSTING

The integrity that is so attractive is also maddening. Indigos hold the rest of us up to the same level of effortless, inborn alignment. They can actually be really impatient and short-tempered with others. They hold us to their standard because, for them, being able to trust others is the only way they can relax enough for intimacy to develop. They inevitably have to wait a long time, because no one else naturally has this gift.

For most of us, living true to ourselves is an elusive, lifelong pursuit. The exception to this is: if our intentions are pure, Indigos feel safe around us. Unfortunately, most of us fluctuate in our motives from moment-to-moment. We go from unintentional or cloudy, at best, to manipulative or contrived, at worst. For this reason, Indigos have a difficult time relaxing into most relationships.

Indigos have to take care not to be overly critical of others, especially in their personal relationships. They can assert inappropriate control when they see others being inauthentic. Indigos do not feel happy with themselves when they are critical and controlling. But it is very difficult for them to disconnect from that faultfinding cycle once it has begun.

NEED AUTHENTICITY IN ORDER TO TRUST
For those who wish to help Indigos in their social struggles, the more true we can be to ourselves, the more trust we will earn—no matter what our personality is. Indigos just need authenticity. It is the only way they can relax around other people. It is the only way they can gauge or make sense of relationships.

The more we manipulate, accommodate, control, mimic and morph ourselves, the less Indigos like us, trust us, or want to be around us. It is as if they "will" us to be true. On the flip side, it is also important for Indigos to show patience and understanding toward the differences they see in others.

JUDGMENTAL
Indigos can go into heavy judgment about others, throwing out people and even whole institutions because of the integrity fluctuations of the individuals within them. An Indigo is drawn to truth, but sometimes they will not make the effort to filter through the junk to get to the heart of things. They can be too prideful and arrogant to deal with the insecurities of others, throwing the baby out with the bathwater, as the saying goes.

CONSPIRACY THEORIST TENDENCIES
In fact, uneducated, spiritually dulled, or resistant Indigos find themselves angry at the world; wrapping up in ever increasing theories of conspiracy—about their neighbors, the government, the world, and even those closest to them. They can become renegades and separatists, trusting few, if any other people, and discriminating harshly against most. They resort to "either-or", polarized thinking, and can justify a lot of poor choices in the name of resisting conformity. Of course, they are not the only personalities with this tendency, but they are the most willful and thorough about it. If they are in this mode, one error in a person or an organization will be enough for them to turn their back completely. The danger in this is how much good Indigos can shut out of their lives in the name of willfulness.

IRON WILLS
Indigos have wills of iron. The world had never seen a true iron will until Indigos arrived. No one else is in the same family for willfulness. This strength of will is the power source of their integrity, but it is also a weakness if they do not keep it in check in other areas of their lives.

Contrary to other theories about Indigos, institutional learning can be very refining for Indigos. It helps them understand how they can be part of the larger social culture and adds refinement to their naturally wise, sometimes abrasive souls. Indigos are strong enough and smart enough to take full advantage of what our current institutions offer.

BOUNDLESS MINDS
Indigos do not start off knowing how to convey what they know. Indigo minds are complex and vast, holding many ideas simultaneously, so it can be quite a battle to get the words out in a way that allows others to digest them. But this is necessary for them to bring their wisdom to others.

NEED TO LEARN DELIVERY IN SPEAKING
A big social lesson for Indigos is learning to speak to others. They need to learn parameters around what they say, how much they say, when they should say it, and when enough has been said. They also need to allow space for others to contribute in conversation.

In their teens and into adulthood, Indigos are in a state of downloading all that they know to anyone who will listen. This can be annoying and exhausting for those closest to them but if we keep listening, nuggets of truth will suddenly burst through that can solve major personal and sometimes global problems. The best place for Indigos to learn social rules for communicating, and teaching with clarity, are *within* their families and society's institutions, NOT by separating themselves out from everyone else.

NEED PARAMETERS & STRUCTURE TO FLOURISH

Education can provide parameters, direction and focus that Indigos think they do not want, but actually crave. Contrary to some ideas about Indigos, formal education does not stifle them. Education, in fact, does the opposite for them. It provides points of departure for their brilliant minds. Indigos often know so much more than what they are being taught, but they do not naturally know the structure of relationships. The possibility, for learning to relate to and expand with others, is a part of what formal training offers.

Indigos need education for the truth it can expose them to. But it is essential that they have a good experience with it early on. Then they are willing to filter through the junk to reach truth as they progress through it.

NATURALLY SPIRITUAL & SKEPTICAL

Indigos are naturally spiritual, but they use skepticism as a protective mask. It is their way of a holding out for the absolute truth—the all-encompassing truth that is only found in the mystical experience. Indigos are the deepest of philosophers at heart. They need absolute Truth to exist in this world, and, on a deeper level, they know it does.

RITUALS & MEDITATION LEAD THEM TO GOD

Religion not only provides Indigos with access to profound principles; it also exposes them to pure, personal rituals and practices they long for. The religious life, in its simplicity and purity, greatly appeals to Indigos.

Institutions in general are large and provide a certain anonymity that Indigos crave. They provide them with much needed space where overarching principles and undercurrents of truth can be observed and assimilated by repetition, and over time. If Indigos are committed to religion and spirituality, they allow themselves to be accountable to someone else. They become accountable to God.

NEED GOD—SOMEONE WHO KNOWS MORE
Their willfulness is brought to the forefront most intensely in relationship to God. No one is more challenged by the concept of a supreme Creator, and no one has a greater need for an all-knowing being in which they can completely trust.

As multi-dimensional learners, there are no boundaries around what is possible. The quantum world, a holographic universe or matrix existence are all things easily conceived and inhabited by Indigos. Through the digital revolution of the past decades, we learned that all the boundaries we once thought existed—don't. We watched Indigos push those boundaries away, without even meaning to, just by who they are.

All of these abilities are great and empowering unless they are Godless or without a source. Indigos in communion with God are at peace. Indigos that are not in communion with God are not. They need to feel God's energy encompassing their seemingly limitless thoughts and extending infinitely beyond them. They need to know there is always someone that knows more than they do because, for Indigos, life is a series of encounters with people that know and see far less than them.

EVER IN SEARCH OF BOUNDARIES

If they don't find this connection to God, there is no rest for Indigos. Instead, their minds are running at full power, all of the time, searching, scanning, seeking, and divining, never able to tune out or turn off. They become like a lighthouse whose beacon is trying to reach the edge of the universe.

SINGLE-MINDED IN PURPOSE

Indigos are single-minded in purpose, but without a connection to God it is like they are blindly dropped from a plane at night in a rescue mission. They speed full-throttle ahead, with their will alone as guide, only to find themselves at the edge of a cliff and in the wrong country. This is what figuratively happens to Indigos without God in the details of their lives.

GOD IS THEIR WAY TO BE HELD

A connection to God is like a mother to them; the only place they can curl up into a ball, relax and let go. God is the only place they find a boundary for themselves. Indigos in alliance with their Creator can let go of insecurities and fears, and be the pillars of integrity they came here to be. It is the only path to peace for Indigos.

GIFT OF WISDOM

Like Violets, Indigos are endowed with the gift of wisdom. They are containers of truth. If they are properly self-disciplined within society, and reliant on God, they help us see ourselves as we are and lead us to higher ways of living. If they make efforts toward refinement, and open themselves to the learning and growth that comes from integrating into society, Indigos can positively affect society much more than if they stay on the sidelines.

DOERS & SAYERS OF TRUTH
Indigos are born orators. As containers of truth, they are also mouthpieces for that truth, and we naturally follow their teachings because their lives are congruent with what they teach. Indigos have the opportunity to compound spoken truth, with truth in action, making them the most effective kind of teachers. Indigos lead people to integrity by living their own life in integrity.

PARADIGM SHIFTERS
An educated and spiritually "in-tune" Indigo can affect cultures and the world for good as they pass on enormous volumes of wisdom and perspective to the masses. Indigos shift paradigms. Suddenly we ask, "Why haven't we been doing things like this always?" They lift us up in our collective conscience. They help us rise to the occasion. They do this with their powerful words of truth and with their quiet lives of integrity.

> *"Change will not come if we wait*
> *for some other person or some other time.*
> *We are the ones we've been waiting for.*
> *We are the change we seek."*
> Barrack Obama

SPACEHOLDERS
Indigos hold their own space. They push their own emotional, physical and energetic boundary out as far as they need to. Wherever they push it to, it stays. Indigos are like islands unto themselves. The rest of us comply with their set boundaries or else they do not allow us to be a part of their lives. This rigidity infuriates those closest to them and, in a way, it seems like Indigos are pushing everyone away. In reality, however, they are just holding on to who they are and where they stand at all cost.

If Indigos feel encroached upon by anyone, they will reinforce their borders. Pushing them feels like trying to push through impenetrable steel walls. It simply is not possible. This consistent dynamic is infuriating to others. But, there is method in Indigos' rigidity, conscious or not. Being in relationships with people who will not budge in their identity can serve as a powerful catalyst for others to know and create their own boundaries.

Indigos will always be true to themselves. This stubbornness may actually be their priceless gift to the rest of us. Like steel barges in night waters, wearing down the waves with their effortless persistence, Indigos wear us down until all that is left is what is true about us. All the inauthenticity will crumble away.

INDIGO FAMOUS PEOPLE*
Barack Obama—U.S. President
Bill Clinton—former U.S. President
Matt Damon—actor
Alicia Keys—musician & songwriter
Brandon Boyd—singer, lyricist & artist
M. Night Shyamalan—screenwriter & film director
Mark Zuckerberg—founder of Facebook
Hayden Christensen—actor
Fiona Apple—singer & songwriter
David Wolfe (Yellow)—health expert

*Parentheses signify the secondary part of their main Aura Personality.

~

THE AVENTURINE-CRYSTAL AURA PERSONALITY

The Avatar

"If we find ourselves with a desire that nothing in this world can satisfy, the most probable explanation is that we were made for another world."
C.S. Lewis

HIGH ENERGETIC VIBRATION
Aventurine-Crystals carry a higher energetic vibration than the rest of us, one close to the plane of heaven. Being near them is a brush with eternal truths we all once knew but lost. They embody these irrefutable truths and, if we pay attention when we are near them, they stir something deep within our own infrequently visited, eternal places, reminding us that we were made for something greater beyond this *vale of tears*.

COMPELLED BY ETERNAL PRINCIPLES

Aventurine-Crystals are constantly guided by spiritual principles, even compelled by them. They do not always verbalize about spirituality, but it is in everything they think, energetically extending out from them all of the time.

The fact that we are spiritual beings having a physical experience is most apparent to Aventurine-Crystals. There is a sense that they brought heaven with them. And the heaven they are connected to is active, not passive. In fact, the energy Aventurine-Crystals bring is ecstatic and powerful, mindful and meditative, charged and playful. It is ever changing and interactive, imbued with a compulsion to extend creativity all of the time.

RESTLESS

Aventurine-Crystals have a restless energy about them that, if we define by psychological terms, would be misdiagnosed as Attention-Deficit Hyperactivity Disorder. Or, if we ask them to stay within the bounds of the current education system, we will be responsible for producing a multitude of delinquents, not because anything is wrong with them, but simply because Aventurine-Crystals do not fit any former mold we might use to categorize people or track progress.

Aventurine-Crystals are a new category of human, an unprecedented category. The forerunners that somewhat prepared us for them, at least in terms of behavior and academic performance, are Yellows and Indigos—Yellows because their bodies have so much information running through them at any given time—that sitting, listening and memorizing is a form of torture; and

Indigos because the current education system does not even begin to stimulate their expansive minds.

CREATION & DESTRUCTION ENERGY
As children, Aventurine-Crystals are perceived as extremely physical and distracted. They can look like whirling tornados, spinning and circling around people and objects, leaving physical destruction in their wake. They can be in joy or rage as they race around, frantically trying to come to terms with their bodies and physical, environmental, and social limitations. Aventurine-Crystals are literally bursting with energy.

Where Crystals carry the feeling of angels and peace, Aventurine-Crystals carry the energy of creation and destruction. While Crystals yearn for sanctuary on earth, Aventurine-Crystals are desperately searching for outlets for their dissatisfaction. One of the only ways this dissatisfaction is released is through acts of creation and destruction.

NEED TO ACCEPT BEING IN THE WORLD
Like the other Spiritual Aura Personalities, their acceptance of this mortal world and having a physical body is not automatic because it contrasts with what they know on deeper levels. It feels nothing like what they know to be real. They feel the limitation of the body compared to what is possible. Coming to terms with the various faculties of the body, like emotions, obligations in relationships, and necessary structure, overwhelm them because their natural energy is faster than their sluggish mortal frames can comfortably contain.

EXTROVERTING EXCESS ENERGY

Aventurine-Crystals can be silly, giggly, goofy and active, extroverting as a way to counter all the energy surging up inside of them. The energy of heaven is much more playful than the serious Ego energy we wade around in here on earth. Wide-awake to the whole experience of mortality, their difficulties lie in learning to shut their eyes and rest so that the whole experience of life can be taken in better stride.

ENERGETICALLY FLOODED

If there are no spiritual, intuitive, or feeling languages, dialogues or activities in the home, then what the Aventurine-Crystals do and say may appear very abnormal. With their constant flow of peaking and subsiding energy, they have a couple of ways to vent. One is through absolute outward stillness, the other, constant movement.

Staying physically frozen in place allows the vibrational activity within them to course through. Their bodies become like a barnacle on a stone desperately hanging on while the river rages over, through and around them. They just ride it out, waiting for the surge to ebb.

When Aventurine-Crystals are in this state, their mouths are usually agape and they have the look of someone trying to recall something that has completely eluded them. The interesting thing is that they are present through all of this. They are still able to track what is happening around them. They are just energetically flooded to the point that little or nothing can be expressed.

This experience is similar to the moment of fight or flight when signals from bodily functions, like eating and sleeping, recede into the background. There is a twisting, gridlock experience in the torso that, if described, others might label as anxiety or even distress. But the coursing energy isn't negative, just immense.

ANGELS CONFORMING TO PHYSICAL LIMITS

The second way Aventurine-Crystals experience energy surges is by moving everywhere, all around whatever space they are in, or leaving the situation they are in to head off in a random direction. They just have to go and be on the move. It is very easy to understand what this experience must be like for them if you think of them as former angels, without a mortal body to confine them to laws of gravity and limitations of time.

The Aventurine-Crystals emanate light much larger than their physical frames. They constantly experience the physical aftereffects of that, with bodies limited by pain and grounded by gravity. They know they are truly capable of moving through time and space, and that time and space are relative and insubstantial, so gravity is particularly frustrating for New Spirituals.

> *"It hurts that I can't fly."*
> Cole Bunderson

DISDAIN FOR THE BODY

Aventurine-Crystals have the capacity to see all of us in our light and glory, and acutely feel their own glory, but all of this is transmuted through their physical bodies. They have great difficulty coming to terms with being in a body, seeing it as a great limitation. This is their weakness. The body is not a limitation. The body is a gift. They wanted their bodies. They knew what was possible if body and spirit were combined and, although many of them know this principle, most are not at peace with it.

SOURCES OF RELEASE, EVEN ADDICTIONS
Relaxation, meditation, movement, people, and play are great releases for all of the pent up energy Aventurine-Crystals contain, but they are not sufficient. As they enter teenage years and into adulthood, Aventurine-Crystals seek new possible outlets. It becomes clearer to them that life is an unending search for a place to expand and deposit the energy roiling inside of them. This is when things can get really complicated for Aventurine-Crystals because more and more addictive options are available to them. And addictions bring some relief, albeit temporarily.

CHECKING OUT & REALIGNING
Aventurine-Crystals can mentally and physically check out from the present. Their conscious minds literally take them elsewhere, to places that are nowhere and everywhere.

There is some truth in saying Aventurine-Crystals disconnect when they appear unfocused or mentally absent, but this absence is a bit different from consciously dissociating. Their disconnection is a necessary, impulsive, self-preservation skill that energetically realigns them to what is true.

Aventurine-Crystals find respite in these moments because they step out of mortal time and enter the realm of purely eternal. And, when they return to the room, they are more relaxed and have more clarity than before. The trick is to not use these experiences as a way to escape but, instead, use them to reconnect and fortify their purpose for being here in this world.

> *"Always aim at complete harmony of thought and word and deed. Always aim at purifying your thoughts and everything will be well."*
> Mahatma Gandhi

SELF-DESTRUCTIVE TO COPE WITH ENERGY
The energy coursing through Aventurine-Crystals is spiritual in nature but funneled through the mortal body, so it stirs up and magnifies all the ponderings, passions and sensations of the flesh. That is why there is such an intense instinct to release it in the physical realm. A variety of self-destructive behaviors can manifest when Aventurine-Crystals are unclear about the energy they embody and are too tired to channel it productively.

AWAKE IN A SLEEPING WORLD
Part of their excess energy is a byproduct of being the only ones awake in a world asleep, or having sight in a world of blindness. That solitary knowing-ness of the eternal big picture rankles and agitates, and so they search and search for someone, anyone to understand what it feels like to see so much of what is ridiculous with the world. They have obvious issues with authority because it is difficult to obey someone that compared to you is in the dark, figuratively speaking.

> *Aventurine-Crystals are strangers in a strange land.*

KNOW THE BIG PICTURE, BUT NOT DETAILS
Aventurine-Crystals have no natural patience for the error and destruction they see all around them on earth.

It is very difficult for them to make peace and commit to their own personal life experience amidst such turmoil and unrest.

Aventurine-Crystals know that this life, this world, is a testing ground that is not real or permanent, and that much of what we do is not real or permanent either. They know the eternal realm is what is real. And even though this world is transitory, they sense heaven interacting here and are connected with what is really being played out on earth. What they often forget is the value of being here because the sensory data they channel is so loud and distracting.

When Aventurine-Crystals get a break from their loud energetic systems, they remember the purpose of having this mortal experience. In those moments they experience deep clarity and remind us is that everything is spiritual and good at the core, as is everyone. They remind us that we are missing out on heavenly intervention because of poor choices, and because we disconnect ourselves from the divine. Aventurine-Crystals are here to tell us that what is divine is what is real about us, and the rest is just a mirage that prevents us from seeing that truth.

> *"There are a dozen views about everything until you know the answer. Then there is never more than one."*
> C.S. Lewis

GIFT OF KNOWING

Constantly reevaluating what they believe and why, Aventurine-Crystals want to know how eternal principles apply to their current life experiences. They are in a constant questioning state. On the one hand they know spiritual truth, but on the other they are never settled with finite answers. Aventurine-Crystals are always left wanting more. They have to revisit principles again and again to see what else there is to see. Of course, there is always more to know, but even in knowing there is unrest for Aventurine-Crystals.

Aventurine-Crystals have the gift of Knowing—very different from the spiritual gifts of hope, faith or even wisdom. They just come knowing the really, really big picture. They know from whence we came, and where we are headed. The irony is that they experience constant clarity yet personal peace generally eludes them. This is the trial of Aventurine-Crystals. It is what they must come to terms with in order to access their greatest strengths and finally be able to do what they came to earth to do.

FEARFUL & LONELY IN THE TRUTH
Besides struggling for rest, Aventurine-Crystals are shocked to discover their solitude in sightedness. Their hearts break once they realize most of us prefer blindness to truth and pain to true peace. The rest of us are not worse or less worthy because of our blindness, but we are fools not to trust what Aventurine-Crystals know and try to teach us.

Despite the truth they hold, Aventurine-Crystals are regularly defeated by fear. They fear for the world and for themselves. They wonder how it will all work out. But their greatest fear is that they will not accomplish what they came here to do, which, for them, would negate the purpose of their existence. Mistakes weight heavily on Aventurine-Crystals, and perfectionistic belief systems are common for them.

Aventurine-Crystals can be fatalistic in this way, not trusting the natural rhythm of imperfect mortality. A lot of their lives are spent trying to be a part of this pacing without losing the heaven within them.

MUST NOT SURRENDER

The work for Aventurine-Crystals is to not give up. Their being here is monumental. Their presence alone is a gift the world has rarely experienced before. Although they will not find purpose in the routines and things the rest of us adhere to, they can work beside us and find peace in the routines of life, and satisfaction in relationships with others and with God.

> *"Compassion is*
> *the radicalism of our time."*
> Dalai Lama VIX

GIFT OF COMPASSION

Aventurine-Crystals feel great compassion for all of humanity, but they do so one-by-one. They need to spend time with others for this gift to amplify, but once they do they see heaven easily within others and are able to share it with them.

Aventurine-Crystals offer a grace and acceptance from their hearts when they spend time with others. That experience is so sweet and pure that the receivers get a true glimpse of God's compassion for them and from there begin to remove erroneous self-perceptions.

People feel identified around Aventurine-Crystals. Aventurine-Crystals seem to hold up a mirror that is closer to what God sees than what anyone else has ever seen in them before, including themselves. It is an amazing experience to be truly seen.

Aventurine-Crystal ♦ THE AVATAR

> *"Compassion asks us to go where it hurts,*
> *to enter into the places of pain,*
> *to share brokenness, fear, confusion, and anguish.*
> *Compassion challenges us to cry out with those in misery,*
> *to mourn with those who are lonely, to weep with those in tears.*
> *Compassion requires us to be weak with the weak,*
> *vulnerable with the vulnerable, and powerless with the powerless.*
> *Compassion means full immersion in the condition of being human."*
> Henri J.M. Nouwen

The trick for Aventurine-Crystals is not to let the immensity of compassion they feel towards others confuse them about its source or its purpose. Hormones and cultural views of cloud the purpose of compassion, so relationship boundaries are understandably hazy for Aventurine-Crystals, as well as for those they serve. But they do not have to be. Aventurine-Crystals just always need to know their own intentions. When their sole intention is for others to feel God's compassion, then it is clear; when they are trying to get their own needs for love met by extending compassion to others, then it is not clear. Aventurine-Crystals have a learning curve with this powerful gift, but they deserve love and compassion as well.

Aventurine-Crystals also need compassion extended to them. Their hearts break when they realize that others cannot hold up the same mirror of compassion toward them. They easily get lost in others' details and agendas and resent not being seen by others. Aventurine-Crystals often retreat from relationships when they realize that compassion will not be reciprocated to the degree that they can extend it.

Another Aventurine-Crystal will be the only one able to match their level of compassion, similar to how thoughtfulness can only be fully reciprocated from one Blue-Amber to another. But, all close, genuine relationships are vital for Aventurine-Crystals as they explore this life experience and learn to accept mortality. They are social beings that need a lot of love, acceptance and interaction. Giving compassion may be innate for them, but learning to trust others is vital.

MULTI-DIMENSIONAL MULTITASKERS
Aventurine-Crystals are watchful and focused even when they do not appear to be. They are the true multitaskers. Because so much is going on for them internally it is a miracle they can function at all externally. No one else compares to them in this way. Aventurine-Crystals take in so much sensory, energetic and mental information simultaneously that it manifests by some pretty funny body language. They will appear frozen, with a blank or look on their faces, or a distracted one with eyes darting every which way, or their bodies moving all about the room.

These are just a few of the passive ways they shed extra energy. And, despite appearances, Aventurine-Crystals are actually able to catch nearly everything going on around them even when they appear to be daydreaming.

So much is going on energetically for Aventurine-Crystals that it is difficult for them to give focused attention to others, but they are capable of it. They do not need to focus long to experience complete compassion for someone else, but when they do their focus is total.

PLAYFUL, ACTIVATING POWER

Aventurine-Crystals extend a lot of active, playful energy. People feel happy and playful around them. They are natural joy-givers and their playfulness is a great compliment to their depth. Others find themselves giggling more and even moving their bodies more when they are around Aventurine-Crystals.

This playful energy could also be called an activating power. There is a fast-moving energy around them. They are instigating movement in everyone just with their presence. But this activating power is coming from unassuming Aventurine-Crystals, so it is an interesting phenomenon to say the least. Some questions to answer are: What are they activating in us? What are they activating us to do, or where are they activating us to go?

PING-PONG ENERGY

The energy Aventurine-Crystals carry causes them to Ping-Pong into different states. In one moment they are laser-focused on what someone is saying. The next moment they are watching an activity. In another instant they are withdrawn into a sort of trance riding through overactive chakras. Then they are moving all over the room, going outside and coming back in. And before you know it, they are suddenly in their car and driving away.

Aventurine-Crystals seem to live by an internal intuition that tells them what state should have activated at any given time. The clock is completely irrelevant to them. They do whatever they feel to do, moment-to-moment. Of course this makes it very difficult to follow schedules or routines, or fulfill expectations from others. But who is to say they should cease listening to their intuition and their energy? Maybe we should all be listening and following it?

CANNOT GO AGAINST WHAT THEY KNOW
Like Indigos slowing us down to a natural rhythm, Aventurine-Crystals are shifting us into heavenly energy. They are interrupting the unnatural frenzy of society. They do not abide the frenzy and step to the side of it.

Also like Indigos, Aventurine-Crystals can be misread as antisocial because of this, but that is a sad misunderstanding of who they are. They are not antisocial; they are just choosing not to participate in meaningless activity. Aventurine-Crystals are incapable of going against themselves in order to join the futile, warring, ridiculous, Ego-driven way we live. For them to do so would be like chopping down a tree and still expecting the limbs to bear fruit. Besides being absurd, it is simply outside the realm of possibility for Aventurine-Crystals to participate in detrimental or needless activities.

UNKNOWABLE
Aventurine-Crystals feel unsure of their behaviors and actions, whether or not they are socially acceptable, but they do not experience a fundamental self-doubt because of this awareness; they are just often lonely. Aventurine-Crystals are not fundamentally insecure, like Crystals, they just feel unidentified and adrift, more like Indigos.

TIME IS MEANINGLESS
Aventurine-Crystals appear intellectually slow at times, but they are most certainly not. Their pacing is just naturally attuned with the spiritual, the eternal instead of with the clock. Aventurine-Crystals actually run faster

than the rest of us, energetically speaking. Time is of no meaning for Aventurine-Crystals, or any New Crystals. They play with time, in fact, and perceive it as an interesting game and pointless phenomenon.

LESSONS IN THE PHYSICAL REALM
Most of us have to remind ourselves to practice our spirituality and religious duties. In stark contrast, these Aventurine-Crystals need reminders to do the mundane physical and mental tasks of life. Many Aventurine-Crystal lessons are within the physical plane. Their eternal, expansive spirits need to conform to limited bodies, minds, voices and emotions so they can learn the lessons that only come from this union. But the shift into mortal life is difficult for them, difficult to tame the energy surging within them and still hold on to their spiritual missions.

SAD THAT WE ARE IGNORANT
Aventurine-Crystals are connected to heavenly energy but they can be hopeless, disappointed in God, and unsure about what He is asking of them. They want to feel more peace in their existence, but their primary questions for God are about the rest of us.

We are all very frustrating and ignorant-appearing to Aventurine-Crystals, but instead of feeling superior about this, they feel sorrow. Our lost and fallen state is the thing apparent to them about all of us. In their sight, we are like too many ants in a small space, bumping into each other, constantly backpedaling because we cannot find a clear path or leader to follow. Our spiritual blindness is blatantly obvious to Aventurine-Crystals and they feel sorrowful watching us struggle in darkness when the light is so clear to them.

Aventurine-Crystals are sad in a detached way. Their sorrow is not emotional but involves a sense of grief and loss too deep for tears, one entwined in the energetic fabric of existence before we came here and where we are headed after. They have difficulty finding a context for these deep feelings of grief. Aventurine-Crystals have to really watch their tendency for hopelessness and despair and remember that they are needed and wanted on earth.

> *"(Frodo) I wish the ring had never come to me.*
> *I wish none of this had happened.*
>
> *(Gandalf) So do all who live to see such times.*
> *But that is not for them to decide.*
> *All we have to decide is what to do*
> *with the time that is given to us."*
> From *Lord of the Rings*, by J.R.R. Tolkien

LONELY BEING AWAKE

Aventurine-Crystals are lonely in their Knowing. It is like we are part of a matrix and they are the only ones on the outside looking in, the only ones aware of the multiple dimensions. The rest of us rarely if ever cross over into that eternal space with them. When we do, they feel such great relief for the company that they finally share openly the spiritual truths they hold. These brief, infrequent encounters with us are where Aventurine-Crystals experience their purest joy. It provides them with a glimpse that everyone else is not lost, and it allows them a moment to feel seen and known.

TRULY CONSCIOUS & FULLY PRESENT

Aventurine-Crystals have the opportunity to model to the rest of us what being fully in the present and fully awake to life looks like. It feels amazing to be in the present moment with someone for them because that is one of their missions.

Aventurine-Crystals are here to teach us that the past is nothing, the future does not exist, and all that is real is the present. The present is uncluttered consisting of us, and our connection to heaven in any given moment. True peace resides in their kind of present. Aventurine-Crystals live in the present far more than anyone else and they wish the rest of us would join them.

Aventurine-Crystals are some of the only people that can consistently follow through with impressions, promptings and intuition. They are meant to live guided by light and inspiration on a continual, moment-to-moment. That is the only way they feel at peace in this world. Living fully in the present is the way to true consciousness. Although they are judged for being attention-deficit, Aventurine-Crystals need to take most of their steps via promptings.

> *"To become more conscious is the greatest gift anyone can give to the world."*
> From *Power Vs. Force*, by David R. Hawkins

WORDS & CONFIDENCE

Aventurine-Crystals are confident. This confidence inevitably triggers the rest of our Ego-driven minds, but Aventurine-Crystals are simply confident in what they know and have a difficult time understanding why everyone is not equally confident. The rest of us find it difficult to relate to such clear intentions, or to people so internally driven by heavenly vibrations.

Their confidence often approaches arrogance. Aventurine-Crystals become resistant to others easily.

Their minds are sometimes so focused on their own agendas that others cannot say anything right for them. Aventurine-Crystals have to take care not to be critical in their verbal interactions.

Speaking feels particularly slow to Aventurine-Crystals. Others cannot speak fast enough for them. They feel impatient in listening, but also in speaking, frustrated that all they experience, in so many dimensions, has to be reduced to the spoken word. Due to these frustrations, Aventurine-Crystals have the makings of becoming quite gifted writers and orators.

LEAD US INTO ETERNAL
If we let them, Aventurine-Crystals trail-blaze us toward light. They step us into the rhythm of the eternal and out of the chaotic nonsense of the ego-driven, self-destructive world. Seeing without effort through eyes of compassion, Aventurine-Crystals restore our sight to who we really are and how valuable we really are.

> *"As you care less about*
> *what people think of you,*
> *you will care more about*
> *what others think of themselves."*
> Stephen R. Covey

~

THE MAGENTA-CRYSTAL AURA PERSONALITY

The Saint

"For as the heavens are higher than the earth, so are my ways higher than your ways, and my thoughts than your thoughts."
From *The Book of Isaiah: 55:9*

SLOWED RHYTHMS
Magenta-Crystals are a bit like planets unto themselves, rotating on axes in their own solar systems, on their own planes, each at their individualized speeds as they go through the cycles of life. There is a sense of constancy, strength and order to them, but also a distinct separateness.

They seem almost untouchable. The world can be in chaos, but Magenta-Crystals stand apart. They are reminiscent of sea turtles in routine, durability, speed and longevity. Nothing will interrupt their rhythms. Like sea turtles, Magenta-Crystals need an internal space as vast as our world's oceans to workout their minds and actualize their purposes. If they do not learn how to provide for themselves, then life is experienced as constant turmoil.

Magenta-Crystals are on a journey to live true to their rhythms and have the world support them in that, instead of the reverse. They are sometimes called lazy and irresponsible, and oftentimes wonder if those labels are true because compared to the external behavior of others, their way of life looks lazy.

Magenta-Crystals spend a lot of time daydreaming, doing tasks or hobbies that interest them, thinking, meditating and sleeping. Compared to the rest of us their natural rhythm feels slowed down by days filled with such introspective activities. But Magenta-Crystals cannot be busy just for busy-nesses sake. Busy-ness, of itself, is meaningless to them. Like all New Crystals, there must be a larger purpose in all that they do. Neither completing tasks nor following traditions meet that requirement.

ALPHA MIND STATE
One Magenta-Crystal woman described feeling like she spent most of her time in an alpha state of mind (which is an apt description of what Magenta-Crystals feel like to other people). The alpha state is a highly relaxed mind-state that leaves the body feeling restive and peaceful. When our minds are operating at an alpha

brainwave frequency, they are highly receptive—the state we are in when we passively watch television, drive a car on a known route, or gaze at lights on a Christmas tree.

Operating primarily from this relaxed mind state, Magenta-Crystals create lives and behaviors to support it, spending hours and days to themselves. Others may occupy the same space, but it is as if Magenta-Crystals are in a dimension too far away to notice.

*"I check out, but really
I'm just checking in."*
Shannon Davis

IRRITABLE & SELF-ABSORBED

Living primarily in an alpha-state, Magenta-Crystals feel like they are getting woken up or interrupted by others. It is understandably easy for them to view people, and any outside stimuli for that matter, as irritants. For the rest of us it would be like someone asking us questions while we are trying to watch a movie, constantly tugging us in and out of separate mind-states.

Magenta-Crystals react to alpha-state interruptions from others by isolating themselves from others or overreacting to them. Magenta-Crystals do not like charged emotional exchanges, so they develop an alternate strategy. They master control of whether or not communication happens with others at all.

This can be fairly difficult limitation for loved ones and prohibits closeness but happens because of how overwhelmed and absorbed Magenta-Crystals can become in their thoughts and the energetic realm. If they are working through something, everything else is seen as intrusion, including people.

Those close to Magenta-Crystals have to try not to get consumed. Magenta-Crystals are powerful and others fall easily into their powerful, sedating rhythms. When that happens it feels like their world is the whole world. Because the risk of losing your sense of self is so high with them, the potential to find it is equally high. Magenta-Crystals are unintentionally persuasive, but they actually need and prefer others to hold onto their own perspectives around them. Objectivity serves as an anchor to Magenta-Crystals while they travel different energetic realms and they really appreciate people who offer it.

Magenta-Crystals do not want to be so isolative or so controlling in their relationships, they just do not know how to involve people in their inner worlds and still feel safe. They have to follow their own rhythms but they would love companionship along the way, and the opportunity to find a context for their gifts and the clear, powerful energy they emanate.

Some very intuitive parents, of a 2-year-old Magenta-Crystal, are already practicing taking the lead with their daughter when she is in that separate, alpha state. They recognize her need to control her environment by separating out but they have realized she also wants them to enter her realm with her and even lead her in it at times.

Magenta-Crystals are very vulnerable in the alpha state it is no wonder they isolate much of the time. But as they try to achieve a sense of safety in being who they are, they need to realize that other people can be a part of their world and that give-and-take relationships are possible while still maintaining personal space and inner congruence.

DISCIPLINED
Actions and thoughts are very controlled for Magenta-Crystals. There is a discipline in them that, if not innate, is rapidly and thoroughly learned and implemented almost all of the time.

The minds of Magenta-Crystals are a vast expanse yet they tend to hyper-focus on one thing at a time, gathering all that they can until they have reached mastery of that thing. It is like they consume chunks of knowledge in huge gulps. Science, physics, metaphysics, history, philosophy and religion are like bedtime stories to them. Their minds love the broad expanse of knowledge that is infinitely ongoing in possibility. Each area pacifies their yearnings to know, but only momentarily. Magenta-Crystals have minds incapable of stopping a thought once it starts. Their minds are like the expanse of the universe, similar to Indigos and other Spiritual Aura Personalities.

With their bright minds, Magenta-Crystals have an almost childish faith that leaves them vulnerable and devastated by reality, and angry at the inconsistencies and incongruities. But part of their lessons, part of their journey here is to pass from childish faith into childlike faith.

Their faith has to refine for it to continue serving them, or else they are just continually let down by their perception of God's role in their life and the actions and words of others.

AURA PERSONALITIES

> *"When I was a child, I spake as a child,
> I understood as a child, I thought as a child:
> but when I became a man, I put away childish things."*
> From *The New Testament*,
> by Paul to the Corinthians (1 Cor. 13:11)

SELF-CONTAINED

Magenta-Crystals have an instinctive ability to get themselves back into a relaxed state when it has been disturbed, or when others are stressed; they find a way to disconnect from it. For example, a personality consultation with a family was definitely hovering at beta brainwave frequencies of stress and high engagement. The parents were frustrated, wanting their Spiritual Aura children to have the same social acceptance and integration they experienced as Mental and Body Aura Personalities. At some point in the discussion, the 9-year-old Magenta-Crystal son had assumed and maintained the lotus position and was in self-imposed meditation. The mom shrugged it off, saying "He just does weird stuff like that sometimes."

Rather than being "weird stuff" however, being able to quickly shift into an alpha mind state is actually an amazing ability of Magenta-Crystals. They naturally, unconsciously know how to induce relaxation in themselves and in others. They can improve this ability with practice, and are interestingly drawn to activities that encourage meditative states, but the talent is innate.

MIND POWER & MINDFULNESS

Not everyone appreciates the way they feel around Magenta-Crystals. This sedating effect can feel unnerving—like a loss of control, to some degree. Magenta-Crystals can make others feel uncomfortable without either party understanding that this is the reason why.

Staying alert and on-edge is the way some people choose to live, but Magenta Crystals can throw that off with their sedating energy. It can feel like the martial arts technique of swiping the air directly in front of your opponent's body before going in for an attack. Many of us are not used to believing we are safe enough to be relaxed, so we wrongfully confuse the relaxing feeling Magenta-Crystals induce with the belief that they are unsafe. It is unfortunate that we have become a society that mistrusts the very people who could teach us how to achieve personal peace.

Most of us do not know how to access the peace that lies within us so we often depend on repetitive, external stimuli to induce relaxation. We irresponsibly expose ourselves to things like television that have the same effect as Magenta-Crystal energy of dropping our brains into alpha state where we are physiologically relaxed and mentally receptive, but instead of feeding us truths, it fills us with endless, repetitive, morally neutral, and sometimes degrading propaganda.

This does not mean we should allow the next Magenta-Crystal we meet to hypnotize us, but it does mean that we are far more likely to experience inner tranquility and intuitive ideas in their presence than by watching a few hours of television.

Magenta-Crystals have an incredibly high moral compass, directing all that they say and do, powerful enough to subdue the temptations that are side effects of being able to influence people on a subconscious level.

But consistent watchfulness is necessary as well, as there is potential for abuse or irresponsibility. Magenta-Crystals will have to repeatedly demonstrate their high moral character in order to gain the trust of others as well as fully develop and utilize this extraordinary gift.

PEACE FROM THE INSIDE OUT
There is no such thing as pushing Magenta-Crystals into action. They will not budge. Their pace does not vacillate. Magenta-Crystals are mostly passive but there is a push in their energy as well, a constant, rhythmic, unhurried push, like an iceberg carving its way through rock leaving giant canyons in tow. Magenta-Crystals are slowly, consistently carving their way into our subconscious minds, shifting us into mindfulness and personal responsibility, causing significant metamorphosis in our collective consciousness, reminding us that peace on earth comes from within.

Magenta-Crystals are affecting change with their innate mindfulness and presence. They have an ability to disengage from conflict and become centered and peaceful, regardless of what goes on around them. Magenta-Crystals are teaching us by example how to be stewards of ourselves, moving the world toward peace by working within themselves and, unknowingly, extending that peace outward to the rest of us.

In many ways their peaceful detachment might be perceived as apathy, but it is far from. Their detachment is actually high personal accountability and personal integrity. When there is conflict they instinctively draw inward and center themselves in stillness. That is one of their main gifts to give the world.

> *"Make peace with silence,*
> *and remind yourself that it is in this space*
> *that you'll come to remember your spirit.*
> *When you're able to transcend an aversion to silence,*
> *you'll also transcend many other miseries.*
> *And it is in this silence that*
> *the remembrance of God will be activated."*
> Wayne W. Dyer

RELATIONSHIPS OR SOLITUDE

There is a learning curve with detached mindfulness. The obvious weakness at the other end of the spectrum is disconnecting from people altogether. An understanding of this ability, and its inherent strengths and weaknesses, is necessary for all the people in the lives of Magenta-Crystals.

It is easy to see how detachment will detract from relationships even being possible for them. Magenta-Crystals need to learn how to disengage while simultaneously maintaining relationships of clear communication and intimacy. This dynamic can work with people who support disengagement as a positive ability, and not as a weakness.

Magenta-Crystals do not need relationships for the sentimental and traditional reasons others need them. They are not sentimental, and are far from being considered traditional but, like many of us, they need them for support.

Relationships with Magenta-Crystal can feel quite neutral to the other party. The object of the relationship is symbiosis, not high romance or dependency. Magenta-Crystals do not feel the same kind of pressing need for romance that many of the rest of us feel. They are fairly self-contained. Significant others serve as essential anchors for Magenta-Crystals as they travel to other dimensions via silence, rituals, sleep, prayer, contemplation or meditation. Loved ones are touch points to everyday reality, and Magenta-Crystals appreciate that kind of commitment and constancy above all else in their relationships. Closeness with Magenta-Crystals happens over time in a relaxed, natural way once they realize they will still have all the room they need to be true to their energy.

FASTIDIOUSNESS & PERFECTIONISM
Because they feel so lost in the realm of relationships, Magenta-Crystals work hard on themselves in hopes of becoming infallible. If they become infallible, then others will not leave, they believe. But their high standard of perfection places them out-of-reach of others. It takes a lot of energy to be fastidious. Suddenly if others cannot support their fastidious behaviors, then there is no room for them. The behavior Magenta-Crystals adopt in order to draw companions to them is the very thing that pushes them away. Magenta-Crystals have to take care not to push companionships right out of their lives with perfectionistic tendencies.

As with all Spiritual Aura Personalities, Magenta-Crystals experience their greatest challenges in the realm of relationships. They also learn and grow the most within the context of relationships. Many of their gifts and talents manifest effortlessly in the realm of energy, but the way those gifts that can develop within relationships are exponentially greater in effect.

MONOGAMOUS & LOYAL

Despite their reserved natures, Magenta-Crystals love companionship. They need soothing and consistent physical touch. Like the other Spiritual Aura Personalities, touch helps them feel less conflicted about their physical bodies and connects them more fully to the earth and other people.

Magenta-Crystals carefully choose one person at a time to partner with, whether that is a parent, a peer or a lover. They will single out someone and then expect constant companionship. However, those companions must be malleable, willing to follow the lead and live within the timeframe of Magenta-Crystals for the relationship to work because Magenta-Crystals will always choose solitude over pairing with inflexible companions. Magenta-Crystals do best with doting friends and companions that will never leave them, no matter how much space or special consideration Magenta-Crystals need.

Magenta-Crystals acutely feel the ongoing growing pains of their metamorphosis through life—learning to manage their vast hearts and powerful energy fields so that they can give of themselves productively to the world. They also know that those closest to them experience their growing pains symbiotically. For that, Magenta-Crystals are extremely grateful for those willing to stay the course with them, no matter how tumultuous it gets, and give generously of themselves to those companions.

> *"The glory of friendship is…*
> *the spiritual inspiration that comes to one*
> *when he discovers that someone else believes in him*
> *and is willing to trust him."*
> Ralph Waldo Emerson

AUTONOMY & AN INTERNAL CLOCK

Magenta-Crystals are moving us toward autonomy with their self-maintained lives of simplicity and centeredness. They are silently demonstrating to the rest of us that we are being dictated to by social constructs, and they are not. We may be angry at them for not going at our pace, but it is futile. Their way is congruent with nature; they are simply following an internal clock connected to universal rhythms. Trying to stop it would be like trying to interrupt the migratory pattern of whales by dropping a pebble in the ocean.

SCARCITY VS. SIMPLICITY

Magenta-Crystals naturally streamline and downsize on their road to autonomy. The less they feel compelled to take part in our capitalist society, the more difficult it is for them to work for income. Magenta-Crystals love simplicity and clarity within and outside of themselves, and materialism is not conducive to that. But Magenta-Crystals also like comfort, so it can be a bit of a quandary finding balance between having a comfortable environment and stepping away from materialism. Simplicity can trigger a scarcity mentality for them and is a learning curve for them to sort between the two.

Magenta-Crystals bring to mind ancient cultures where traits like reflective wisdom and simplistic living were encouraged and supported. If someone served in an advisory role, then the responsibility to provide sustenance would be assigned to others. Perhaps Magenta-Crystals are reminding us of that kind of collaborative and cooperative living with their inability to participate in our capitalist ways.

FEELING MISPLACED
Magenta-Crystals prefer not to draw attention to themselves for doing things differently. It is not their intention to be unique. They subtly look for ways to authentically share themselves without making waves, but if they cannot, they easily feel ostracized and find a backdoor out of what they deem to be unwelcoming environments and relationships. Magenta-Crystals are sensitive to how others respond to them and, unfortunately, isolation is often their first solution.

There is no mistaking the energy of Magenta-Crystals. Once you know what it feels like, you cannot miss it. They have a presence that is both quietly powerful and weighted, like elders or sages from ancient tribes. From young ages they experience a sense of not fitting into our current culture. Like many of us they do not like feeling separate, but they are unable to fake closeness in a society that breeds separateness.

In their separateness they often seek for Home, in a universal sense of the word as somewhere out there, somewhere even beyond our realm. Although much of their detachedness is a process of getting into a state of peace, it does not mean they are at peace. Magenta-Crystals look far and wide for peace. They turn to other people, other cultures, the universe, but ultimately only find it when they travel the full distance to that vast quiet places within themselves. As Magenta-Crystals go inward, the rest of us are able to partake of that peace with them.

BROKEN-HEARTED

The journey to the heart is round-trip for Magenta-Crystals. They start from the heart but travel quite far quite fast from that core. As children they experiment with heart energy, their own and others. In their alpha state they check the emotional climate in a room, in people around them, within their own bodies. They maneuver quite easily with the heart. They remind those around them that love is expansive, the heart unlimited. It is child's play to join their hearts to ours. They come with fully mature hearts; unlike anybody we have seen on this planet before.

> *"Our daughter locks herself in our hearts.*
> *She is able to do that not just with us*
> *but with other people as well."*
> Shannon Hansen

But what they find out quickly is that most of our hearts are not open, that we use them as battlegrounds instead of gateway for peace. Magenta-Crystals are devastated by this misuse and abuse.

In the shock of our collective heart dysfunction, Magenta-Crystals buy into the victim-mode that everything is happening to us and we cannot change the chaos. Because Magenta-Crystals feel so much in their hearts, including all the messiness of life, irresponsibility in relationships with others, and ourselves, and even what we are doing to our planet, that they surrender their heart powers. Their intuitive heart knowledge shifts into a belief that feelings are overwhelming and unmanageable—too much sensation, too much pain—and so their minds race to find refuge.

In the process of escape from feeling too much, Magenta-Crystals overdevelop their minds, finding maneuverability in knowledge. Knowledge becomes their place of power. They also master other areas, tending to dominate their bodies, behaviors, and even their relationships. Magenta-Crystals can get to the point where they completely detach from knowing their own hearts and residually stop feeling the hearts of others as well. This is partially why other people become unknowable to them and relationships become their scariest arena.

This experience is very different from the emotional-connectedness Blues experience in relation to their own hearts and the hearts of others. Magenta-Crystals hearts are sentimental like Blues but they feel their loud hearts more like children experiencing complex emotional intricacies without context or understanding. Early on they see this aspect of themselves as a huge liability and something to extinguish, if possible.

ABUNDANT HEARTS ON FIRE

Despite their efforts to put out the fire in their hearts, Magenta-Crystals always experience a dull, ongoing ache that they do not know how to navigate or manage. At moments they feel so much in their hearts that, if they could, they would lie facedown on the earth, open a doorway to their chest cavities and let the excess energy rush out of them into the earth. The energy feels torrid, immense, unknowable and overactive.

Interestingly, this heart energy is their core, their thing, their gift, what they are really all about. It is not a thing to be feared but cultivated. In all of their quiet, alpha meanderings, the heart serves as the generator, acknowledged or not.

The heart is not a terrifying, out-of-control, raging emotional monster. It is actually quite simple, straightforward and clear compass for a truly peaceful journey through life. Meditation, prayer and communing in nature are gentle entry points for Magenta-Crystals to remember that.

LOVE OF GOD
Magenta-Crystals love deeply and are deeply loved. If you go in with them, it will probably be for the long haul but it is well worth the cost because, occasionally, some of their endless heart energy will pour into your heart. Once you have experienced that, you will know that there is almost nothing like it in this world, because it is not of this world.

If they are worthy and in integrity, Magenta-Crystals are capable of giving love akin to the love of God. It is a love so pure, vulnerable and intense that you will never want it to leave, but we do not need to fear that because it is a lie to think that love is scarce. Magenta-Crystals know this. They are capable of lighting our hearts on fire with a love that cannot be extinguished. It is love that is not attached to false limiting beliefs of scarcity or selfishness.

Magenta-Crystals are blind to this capacity within themselves but, once they remember it and relearn how to extend it to others, it becomes one of the most generous gifts imaginable.

> *"He who binds to himself a joy*
> *Does the winged life destroy;*
> *But he who kisses the joy as it flies*
> *Lives in Eternity's sunrise."*
> William Blake

Magenta-Crystals are learning, slowly but surely to overcome their fears and unlock the floodgates of their hearts so love can pour forth. They have not had role models to demonstrate this, but once they figure it out, watch out world because love will overflow. We thought we knew how to love, but Magenta-Crystals are showing us the abundant way, the kind of love that will never run out. That coupled with their peaceful energy can usher us into a world of true unity.

~

AURA PERSONALITIES

THE AMETHYST-CRYSTAL AURA PERSONALITY
The Angel

"Bring peace to the Earth by bringing peace to all those whose lives you touch. Be peace. Feel and express in every moment your Divine Connection with the All, and with every person, place, and thing.

...Be a living, breathing example of the Highest Truth that resides within you. Speak humbly of yourself, lest someone mistake your Highest Truth for boast. Speak softly, lest someone think you are merely

calling for attention. Speak gently, that all might know of Love. Be a gift to everyone who enters your life, and to everyone whose life you enter…I HAVE SENT YOU NOTHING BUT ANGELS."
From *Conversations With God,* By Neale Donald Walsch

INNOCENT & WISE
Amethyst-Crystals simultaneously carry traits of innocent children and wizened adults. They are bright, kind and forgiving, yet cultivated and experienced. From their sweet demeanors we also sense they know more than the rest of us, even when they are young. They are like J.R.R. Tolkien's Elven race in *The Lord of The Rings,* simultaneously ancient and youthful. Because of this, they seem to experience the tragedies and all the happenings of our world from a distance, aware but somehow a step away from personal involvement. It is like they have seen it all before.

> *"…perhaps all our earthly trials will appear foolish to us after a while; perhaps they seem so now to angels."*
> From *Wives and Daughters,* By Elizabeth Gaskell

For the most part, the things that tempt the rest of us do not tempt Amethyst-Crystals. They do not judge the rest of us for our poor choices, but they do have a difficult time understanding why we do anything with ill intent in mind. That does not mean Amethyst-Crystals never hurt other people, but it is never their intention. Their temptations reside at the soul level; their battles are primarily internal.

NEUROSES AS DISTRACTION

Amethyst-Crystals have heighted nervous systems, similar to Crystals, which make them highly sensitive on physical and emotional levels. They are uncomfortable with their sensitivity. They feel susceptible and vulnerable. They view vulnerability as a liability and they afraid of it. They spend a lot of energy worrying about their vulnerabilities and that worry can manifest as anxiety or other neuroses. Amethyst-Crystals do not want others to suspect how vulnerable they feel and try to detract from it by hyper-focusing on illness and problems.

CONSCIOUS WITH BOUNDARIES

If someone needs help, it does not occur to Amethyst-Crystals not to help. They are kind and thoughtful without forethought. They have issues with boundaries when they extend charity—similar to Blue, Lavenders and Crystals. Amethyst-Crystals get lost in the emotions and troubles of others and retreat in order to find themselves again. They even create personal problems as a way to create emotional and physical space away from others.

But Amethyst-Crystals enjoy people too. They plan time to spend with others and all of their friends play a huge priority in their lives. Amethyst-Crystals can be quite playful and silly. They love to help others relax and wonder why we are all not laughing and relaxing more. In fact, they specifically create environments of peace and calm and fun in an effort to serve others.

Although they love peace, Amethyst-Crystals feel the emotions of others and do not like to ignore them, no matter the intensity. It is very important to them that others feel understood. Amethyst-Crystals have a gift for helping others identify and work through their feelings. They feel more personal peace when they walk through those steps with others. They wish all of us would take the time to care for each other and ourselves in this way.

INDEPENDENCE & PACING
Amethyst-Crystals like to do things on their own and not answer to others, except maybe one other person. They are highly independent. Part of their independence is a way to create physical and emotional space, but the other part is that they are running on their own clock. Amethyst-Crystals, just like all New Crystals, are not concerned with the pacing of our current culture. Something inside them dictates a pacing that is much louder than the call of society.

Amethyst-Crystals have their own unique pace; theirs is a rapid pace. It is not rushed, pushed or intense, it just has a lot of movement to it. Their minds move quickly and their bodies are often in motion to match. Amethyst-Crystals are busy independent individuals. They seem to be involved in some activity or task most of the time.

Different than the other Crystals, however, they do not like to cause a disturbance with their unique pacing. Amethyst-Crystals are one of the most accommodating of all the Spiritual Aura Personalities. They are working out how to be true to their own internal clocks while still considering the needs and pacing of others.

FEAR TO FAITH
Amethyst-Crystals battle with feeling powerless. Like most of us when we feel powerless, they search for ways to exert control. The difference is that they feel much

more anxiety in connection with feeling powerless than the rest of us. They feel terrified and helpless to the point of using desperate methods to gain a sense of control. They will run around trying any kind of remedy to feel peace; these methods and remedies can be helpful, but not always. Sometimes they become addictions. Amethyst-Crystals have to watch themselves in this regard. They need to stop, reflect, and go inward to find the peace they seek, when they find that they are fruitlessly grasping at anything and everything around them.

Amethyst-Crystals have to trust that their unique pacing and their emotional-connectedness to everything and everyone have great purposes. These differences are not things to run or distract from. They feel out-of-control only when these gifts are not seen for what they are.

Amethyst-Crystals often feel lost and out-of-control in this world, but it is no wonder since they are royal angels made for another world. What they have forgotten is that their otherworldliness is needed here and that they are the unique souls to bring heaven to earth. If Amethyst-Crystals can understand and accept this about themselves, they will find the peace and commitment necessary to carry out their missions and help transform our planet.

> *"Faith is not something to grasp,*
> *it is a state to grow into."*
> Mahatma Gandhi

CHILDREN OF CRYSTALS
All New Crystals share many traits with Crystals, but Amethyst-Crystals identify with them the most. They struggle with self-image and self-esteem like Crystals, but

Amethyst-Crystals have an elusive confidence that comes and goes. Sometimes they are immune to the opinions of others, and other times too affected. They feel powerful and confident at times, then suddenly lost and powerless.

PEDESTALED & PROTECTED BY OTHERS

Amethyst-Crystals are like sprites others wish to capture in mason jars and keep near their bedsides for daily doses of heavenly energy, including delight and wonder. Yet they have the same fragile vulnerability as Crystals, and others tend to want to take care of and protect them because of it. They seem rare like diamonds yet fragile like glass. Others worry about them but also admire them for their angelic qualities.

We cannot help but want to simultaneously protect and admire Amethyst-Crystals. We all have a sense that we are in the presence of a rare species when we are with them; that they are like us yet always somewhat separate and apart from us.

Although they are not intimidating, there is something so otherworldly and awe-inspiring about Amethyst-Crystals that others cannot help pedestaling them. Where Crystals seem clueless and gullible, Amethyst-Crystals seem careworn and surrendered. An image of tattered angels readily comes to mind. They have an innate sophistication, refinement and wisdom in them, but have somehow also maintained openness to life and to others. We are lucky and blessed to have their light amongst us.

REMEMBRANCES OF HEAVEN

Part of the mystique of Amethyst-Crystals lies in their remote demeanors. Amethyst-Crystals are inward drawn.

They find it difficult to look people in the eyes because they do not want their sensitivity revealed.

Amethyst-Crystals seem to be looking simultaneously inward and toward heavenly realms and we all seem to be holding our breaths for that moment when they reveal eternal wisdom from those realms. It will not be in words that Amethyst-Crystals bless us, however, but by their presence. They carry a remembrance of heaven that wrenches our souls and we long for the sensation to repeat.

UNUSUAL & CREATIVE
Amethyst-Crystals are sweet but unusual. They do not feel the need to conform but do not like to make waves or cause disturbances by their behaviors. They are not trying to draw attention with unusual behavior; they just feel things more personally and intensely than others, at times, and need to express that in the quickest, most instinctive way, which is often the most unorthodox way. The ways Amethyst-Crystals respond are considered dramatic or even avant-garde to many of us. Luckily they often find socially accepted outlets in the creative arts.

Amethyst-Crystals are drawn to many forms of creativity including writing, drawing, painting, dance and music. They like to be involved in the creation stage of any art form, not just performance. Amethyst-Crystals are able to draw on their emotional and energetic depths. They are inward-focused enough to gestate on ideas until they culminate into profound, raw creations, and those creations are often ongoing in nature, moving and awe-inspiring.

FEEL TOO CONNECTED
Amethyst-Crystals are clever and observant, even though they appear distracted. In fact, they are so connected with and affected by the energy of others that they feel angry with themselves for not being more emotionally available for others. Amethyst-Crystals have consistently loud emotional and energetic voices themselves that vie for attention when they are with others.

There is always so much going on for Amethyst-Crystals internally they often feel they might burst. On the outside it looks like they are ever ready to take flight. With the errand of angels, they never seem to fully relax.

GIFT OF ACCEPTANCE
Despite the belief that they are not giving enough to others, people feel incredible love and peace around Amethyst-Crystals. They exude an unparalleled acceptance toward others and extend instant friendship to all they meet.

There is just a bit of an elusive quality in any relationship with Amethyst-Crystals. They can only give as much as they have to give, which does not always meet up to others' expectations. But what Amethyst-Crystals do give in relationships is so sweet, genuine and pure that it is well worth trading for a little less time or focused attention.

> *"When angels visit us,*
> *we do not hear the rustle of wings,*
> *nor feel the feathery touch of the breast of a dove;*
> *but we know their presence*
> *by the love they create in our hearts."*
> Mary Baker Eddy

ERRAND OF ANGELS

Being around Amethyst-Crystals is like being in the presence of angels. They bring peace, acceptance, love and hope with them wherever they go and with whomever they meet, whether it is a casual encounter or a close connection. Angels are unobtrusive but clear in their purposes. They sing heralds, pronounce, bring comfort and protect. Amethyst-Crystals do the same. They unknowingly have all of these qualities and bring them to the rest of us in the context of a body and within all of their relationships.

Many of the gifts that Amethyst-Crystals give to others are given simply with their presence. They do not need to be at odds with themselves or with what society expects; they just need to understand their unique and specific role as angels, allowing themselves free flight.

Amethyst-Crystals are specifically asked to journey from anxiety to peace, from struggle to victory and, most importantly, from fear to faith. And, if they are able to accept this stewardship, then they have a remarkable opportunity to lead others down the same path, acting as true angels lighting the way.

> *"When you walk to the edge of all the light you have and take that first step into the darkness of the unknown, you must believe that one of two things will happen. There will be something solid for you to stand upon or you will be taught to fly."*
> From *The Leaning Tree*, By Patrick Overton

~

THE INDIGO-CRYSTAL AURA PERSONALITY

The Commander

"Never be afraid to raise your voice for honesty and truth and compassion against injustice and lying and greed. If people all over the world...would do this, it would change the earth."
William Faulkner

COMMANDING CHANGE
Indigo-Crystals bring change; they even force it if others are unwilling to roll with it. They use the megaphone approach to shout us awake to what is going on all around us. They point out the tiniest details that need

change and broadcast dictums for the world at large to correct them.

Indigo-Crystals are brash in their delivery. They move with an energy that shouts, "There's not a moment to lose. Change it, or lose it." Indigo-Crystals keep us on our toes. Just when we think we know something, they authoritatively suggest another way. Like Sergeants, they are keeping us in line, running us through drills, making sure no detail is left unattended. Indigo-Crystals are preparing us for war—a war of souls.

Like a child with an authoritative parent, we resent their delivery, the message and, especially, that it resonates as truth within us. No one wants war, but if it is upon us, will we not prefer to face it rather than be slaughtered from behind because of denial?

Indigo-Crystals do not have the luxury of denying what is. Truth is an active taskmaster for them, and will not let them alone. Their job is to be brash and direct. You cannot wake sedated masses with soothing words; shaking and shouting are in order, and Indigo-Crystals are the ones to do it.

DIRECT IN WORD & ACTION
Unlike the heavy, slow-carving push of Magenta-Crystals, Indigo-Crystals are shoving their way through this world, lightning-fast, equivalent to meteors exploding on contact with the earth's atmosphere, creating instant canyons wherever they land. Indigo-Crystals power-punch clear, direct truths to the minds of anyone and everyone within their reach.

Indigo-Crystals say things that are disarmingly abrupt and direct. They use powerful, succinct and oftentimes very authoritative words without prepping people for the weight of them. Much to their dismay, Indigo-Crystals make people uncomfortable with their directness. This is hard for them to accept about themselves, though most of them are aware of it—it is hard to miss people getting rattled right before their eyes.

> *"It's discouraging to think how many people are shocked by honesty and how few by deceit."*
> Noel Coward

TRANSMITTERS/ORATORS

It takes quite a long time for Indigo-Crystals to learn to speak and teach so that others can receive what they have to say without offense. This is probably one of their most difficult learning curves. Some Indigo-Crystals draw inward as they refine their delivery in speech while others continue to practice on those around them.

People are offended less by content than by delivery with Indigo-Crystals. Although content can be quite abrupt, it is timing and the asking that is often missing in the delivery. They just do not think before they speak. Thoughts come into their minds fully formed and they share them immediately, and fully. Indigo-Crystals are transmitters. Asking them to tone it down, or edit the content would be like intermittently muting a radiobroadcast. We would miss the full message.

FEEL UNAPPRECIATED

Along with timing, it takes a great deal of energy not to act or speak when you intuitively have solutions and answers to the problems around you. Indigo-Crystals are often right in their actions or words, but then overlook clues that people are not always asking for their particular brand of intervention. This is very confusing for them and they can feel like a dog getting kicked for trying to give help.

People need the direct truth that Indigo-Crystals have to give, but they also need to be ready to receive it. Indigo-Crystals have a journey of finding their "spoonful of sugar" to help their truth serum go down a little bit easier.

SOCIAL RULES ELUDE THEM
Social rules elude Indigo-Crystals. Like Indigos, they watch closely for cues but feel frustrated and out of their depth when trying to mirror them, annoyed that such rules even exist. They expend a lot of effort controlling their behaviors, body language and facial expressions in hopes that they are somewhat fitting into normal cultural standards but, as they do so, they remain vigilant to their own truth. They watch for loopholes in the system and, if there is a way to abolish unnecessary social rules, Indigo-Crystals will find it, and liberate the rest of us when they do.

Unlike Indigos, who hideout or cluster in mechanical, techy, or heady realms to avoid mainstream expectations, Indigo-Crystals want to be a part of the masses. They know that their messages are for everyone, not just the minority. As helpless as they feel in navigating social norms, they know they have to figure out how to reach people effectively because their message is vital.

> *"This above all: to thine own self be true, and it must follow, as the night of the day, thou canst not then be false to any man."*
> William Shakespeare

HIGHLY VISIBLE & VULNERABLE
Indigo-Crystals have magnifying energy. When they are in a room, you cannot miss them. They are brash in their words and movements. They are also so mentally present that, speaking or not, their energy is broadcasting loud and clear.

Interestingly, Indigo-Crystals are quite blind to the power and confidence they exude, as well as the effect they have on others. They watch others have strong responses to them but do not understand why. They are literal to the point that they are certain they have missed out on a joke that everyone else is a part of.

EXPERTS & LEADERS
Indigo-Crystals do not know what to do with the strong responses they seem to elicit in others. They feel exposed and quite vulnerable much of the time, like their insides are being worn on the outside of their bodies. Most things feel very personal to them, which make them too subjective to readily evaluate their effect on others.

Interestingly, we look to Indigo-Crystals for leadership, but we also resent them for their power. We ask them for answers and then want them to disappear from our presence.

This dismissive demeanor stems from a society dependent on experts for telling us how to run our lives. We hear them on the television, in books, in lectures, and then we shut off the television, close books and leave lectures. Experts are not people to us. They are simply resources for us to expend and exploit. We use them when we need them, and discard them just as quickly.

Indigo-Crystals come to us with clear knowledge and direct truths. Instead of openly listening to them, and gathering all we can from their light, we flip their switch to silent as we do with any expert, and turn and walk away.

The learning curve for these transmissions of truth is not just for Indigo-Crystals; it is ours as receivers of those transmissions as well. If we do not learn to listen to their direct, honest speech, then we will not be prepared for what will be asked of us in the near future. Indigo-Crystals are here to prepare us; they have been given the marching orders for when we are called to action. They are ready to lead us and they are fully committed to the cause of truth.

> *"The self-confidence of the warrior*
> *is not the self-confidence of the average man.*
> *The average man seeks certainty in the eyes of the onlooker*
> *and calls that self-confidence.*
> *The warrior seeks impeccability in his own eyes*
> *and calls that humbleness.*
> *The average man is hooked to his fellow men,*
> *while the warrior is hooked only to infinity."*
> From *Tales of Power,* By Carlos Castaneda

LITERAL & HONEST

Indigo-Crystals can think symbolically, but prefer words to be used in a straightforward manner. They are literal and honest with their words, using them as a way to navigate trustworthiness in others. This dependency on words leaves them quite vulnerable and gullible, and even makes them susceptible to teasing because they take words so literally.

Indigo-Crystals believe people and hold them to their words. It is difficult for them to understand why anyone would do anything but be direct. Lying is unthinkable for them. They are naturally trusting and often disappointed by people that are more casual with their words.

Alternately, more carefree people often feel pinned to the wall and interrogated when interacting with Indigo-Crystals. Indigo-Crystals will not keep close company long with people they deem frivolous. Being respected, respectable and respect-worthy are high priorities for them and they have a hard time relating with those who compromise those ideals.

All of this is related to Indigo-Crystals' inability to follow social norms unless there is intrinsic value in those norms. Being forthright is the most direct path to truth, where weaving words to open people up to suggestion endows the speaker with a greater capacity to influence and even effect change. Both are possible methods for delivering truth, but the latter requires strategy and subtly. Indigo-Crystals do not do subtly. They will always pick the straightest path to deliver truth and say it thoroughly and outright.

REACTIVE IN RELATIONSHIPS
Indigo-Crystals are easily offended and reactive. They erroneously see many situations as confrontations and easily cause offense with their strong reactions. They are passionate people that try fruitlessly to guard those passions.

Too many interactions feel like natural disasters or calamities to Indigo-Crystals, and to those in relationships with them. They feel immediate remorse for any kind of negative interaction, and their internal compass quickly fills them with regret for acting irritated or being blunt. Self-recrimination moves in so quickly, in fact, that Indigo-Crystals rarely manage apologies. It is quite painful for them to admit that they have offended someone because it is never their intention.

It is difficult for Indigo-Crystals not to feel angry with others for not doing things better, or more truthfully. They have high expectations and are not very rational about those expectations. They can be prideful in their assumptions and unbending in their stances.

Indigo-Crystals experience irritability often and a feeling that nothing is quite the way it should be. They have a hard time not pinning that onto others. But there is a reason why Indigo-Crystals feel a sort of constant discomfort. It is their radar for error so that truth is clearly known when it comes through. Used correctly, this is a powerful tool. But it is not meant as a measuring stick for criticizing others. This is a tricky gift to manage and Indigo-Crystals learn how step-by-step, interaction after interaction.

HYPER-PRESENT & SINGLE-FOCUSED

Indigo-Crystals are focused on delivering truth, so they often forget that not everyone is viewing things from that same paradigm. Some people are focused on the emotional climate, others on the outcome. But Indigo-Crystals have a very difficult time thinking beyond the moment they are in.

Indigo-Crystals have either-or-mentalities. Like their Indigo relatives, they are all-or-nothing in their ideas and lifestyles. They are not middle-ground people. So identifying truth and revealing deceit are always their clearest objectives in every moment, and it is always with pure intention that they do so. Because Indigo-Crystals are so single-minded however, they have a hard time accessing the perspective of others, and conflicts inevitably ensue.

Others experience Indigo-Crystals as fixed and immoveable. Anyone that bumps up against them with their own agenda will get bruised. But Indigo-Crystals also bruise in these collisions. For all their firm, clear words, Indigo-Crystals are surprising softhearted and sensitive. They would like to speak truth and be accepted, regardless of the setting. It hurts them that truth is often unwanted and seen as invasive to others.

LEARN SOCIAL RULES ONE-ON-ONE
Conflict is unfortunately commonplace for Indigo-Crystals and they eventually begin to step back from most relationships after so many. Indigo-Crystals learn early in life that they easily overwhelm others and are often told to tone themselves down. If they are not careful, they start believing that others want them to stop being themselves. "Don't say that," "Tone it down," or "Stop being you," are messages they often internalize.

Some Indigo-Crystals will choose a passive role in a few close relationships, while others will only maintain relationships where they can be completely truthful and true to themselves. This is a safer route for them, but it does not always allow them to extend their truths to others or learn social rules that would help them accomplish that.

However, learning social rules with one person is much easier and safer for Indigo-Crystals than trying to figure out the general rules required for spontaneous interaction with the masses. If they slowly add new relationships into their lives, they can learn the variety of social skills necessary to be able to interact with the masses.

TEACHERLY DEMEANOR
Indigo-Crystals make the most loyal of friends once they know they can trust you and that you love them. But to make the friendship work, you need to allow them to advise you at times. They need to give in this way.

Indigo-Crystals are natural teachers and feel a responsibility to teach those within their association. It is important for them to seek out teaching opportunities so that their close associates do not always feel like they are being lectured. Indigo-Crystals need to teach. It is a significant part of who they are. But they have to learn to do so in contexts where they will actually be received and welcomed for their knowledge.

GUARDED & SERIOUS
Indigo-Crystals' faces match their moods, and their moods are rarely carefree or overtly social. They are not smiley types, similar to Green-Ambers in this way. Indigo-Crystals like people, but because of the intensity of their energy and depth of their thoughts, they can feel standoffish and even antisocial to others. Their literal minds and straightforward manner make for quite serious individuals.

Lighthearted, playful people have a difficult time gauging where they stand with Indigo-Crystals. In turn, Indigo-Crystals are unfamiliar with that type of spontaneous play and generally choose to avoid such companions. This does not mean they never play; they just usually do so with people they know well and trust. Indigo-Crystals do not like unexpected responses from others, and have a difficult time understanding how many of us can open up so quickly and easily with each other.

In some ways Indigo-Crystals feel like they sit on the social sidelines of life and never get a chance to play. This breaks their hearts because they need active and regular engagement with others. Indigo-Crystals are social creatures and the steps they have to take to be part of the game feel like climbing a mountain to them. If they persevere, it is worth it, but they do get tattered and wary along the way. They respond enthusiastically to anyone who extends a helping hand in social settings.

LOST & FOUND
Unbeknownst to the rest of us, Indigo-Crystals vacillate between believing they know-it-all to feeling completely lost. When they are in the lost part of that cycle, they draw inward; when found, they are open and freely impart their knowledge to others.

In one moment they feel full, complete and at peace with the world, the next moment they feel lost, without compass, and filled with regret and guilt without even knowing the cause. It is very hard to take action and move forward in life with such internal contradictions. Indigo-Crystals probably experience ambivalence more than any other Aura Personality.

MORAL COMMANDERS

Indigo-Crystals power is commanding, even instigating. They will usher in monumental change, not by force but by relentlessly broadcasting the error of our ways, and educating us about the actions that we need to take, until we take heed. It is their gift, their job, their mission, and they have to do it regardless of the consequences. Indigo-Crystals want to live truthfully. They want to say what they think and what they know, and they want the same in return from the whole world.

Indigo-Crystals are calling us out. They are uncovering the lies, revealing our lackadaisical demeanors. It is easy to assume they are nit picking, telling us our bed is not made well enough because they cannot bounce a quarter on it, but then we see that they are just saying all of the inadequacies, sparing none. As they speak and speak, revealing our dusty corners and squeaky hinges, our consciousnesses will awake, respond and make the changes that can raise us all to a higher level of existence. Indigo-Crystals are really just our own consciences speaking on the outside of us—they are our Jiminy Crickets. That is why we find them so annoying. If what they are saying is not the truth, we would not be so uncomfortable with it.

> *"Brother stand the pain; Escape the poison of your impulses.*
> *The sky will bow to your beauty, if you do.*
> *Learn to light the candle. Rise with the sun.*
> *Turn away from the cave of your sleeping.*
> *That way a thorn expands to a rose.*
> *A particular glows with the universal."*
> From *Rumi Daylight*, By Mevlana Rumi

Indigo-Crystals' intentions are pure. They do not wish to offend but they do wish to extend truth. They think they are making statements in calm words, but we are experiencing megaphone blasts in the face of direct moral energy from them. Indigo-Crystals are shooting us up with truth serum. The directness grates at our ears, gets under our skin, unveils our hidden attachments to our weaknesses and dependencies but, nonetheless, it is getting in and we are coming out of hiding.

> *"What is to give light*
> *must endure burning."*
> From *Man's Search for Meaning*, By Victor Frankl

∼

THE IMPERIAL TOPAZ AURA PERSONALITY
The Phoenix

"The purpose of life for man is growth, just as the purpose of life for trees and plants is growth. (Man) can grow as he will. ...(Man) can develop any power...Nothing that is possible in spirit is impossible in flesh and blood. Nothing that man can think is impossible. Nothing that man can imagine is impossible of realization."
From *The Science of Being Great,* by Wallace D. Wattles

PHOENIX RISING
Imperial Topazes have the potential to experience pure personal freedom, getting to a place where they do

exactly what they want without forethought and void of regret. But before that takes place, they experience many trials that push them into victimhood to the point that they forget who they are. They forget they ever had any personal power.

Imperial Topazes have a considerable voyage to take before remembering that they are not victims, that power lies within them, and that it cannot be taken from without.

> *"When we are no longer able*
> *to change the situation,*
> *We are challenged*
> *to change ourselves."*
> From *Man's Search for Meaning*, By Viktor E. Frankl

Imperial Topazes have always been on the earth, even though their numbers were down to scores until just recently, but they are metaphorically rising from the ashes in droves, like the mythical Phoenix. They are breaking through their rapid secession of personal trials to emerge as victors, free from the widespread deceit that anything or anyone can limit their growth or hold back their souls.

POWER LIES WITHIN

As a result of the trials they have endured, Imperial Topazes choose to see things as they are. They are fearless about that and know that great harm lies in denying what is. They have no need to view anything through comforting illusion. They know atrocities exist, and although they choose not spend time with negativity they are always willing to take in the whole truth so the most effective and immediate action can come to pass.

Imperial Topazes know that power lies with the individual. To them it is silly to think our fate lies in the hands of any government or individual. It is clear to them that no one thing or person has any real power over us. Imperial Topazes are in the business of reminding us that personal integrity is the only way for us to break free from our individual and collective shackles. They raise people up and out of negativity by introducing them to personal responsibility and accountability.

Imperial Topazes invite life in. They are unafraid of hardship, even abuse, because they know nothing can hurt any of us at our cores. They know we are all sufficiently armored from within to tackle difficulties from without. They know we are equipped to build peaceful internal and external kingdoms from the rubble of our individual and societal wars. Imperial Topazes are excited to let everyone know that rich soil lies beneath all the ashes.

Imperial Topazes can seem unsympathetic to hardship not because they do not see it but because they do not believe in it. Their belief is in what is possible for goodness, wholeness and unity. They always see the bigger picture, a broader landscape where all injustices are viewed as seedlings in plots of fertile soil in the ongoing cultivation process of beautiful humanity.

However cynical we are, however sinister and harmful we believe someone else to be, the truth is that there is a grand unfolding that will benefit all who awaken to their light and actively develop and freely give of their gifts.

IMPERSONAL EMPATHY

Imperial Topazes are empathic like Crystals but, unlike Crystals, the energy of others only sticks long enough to instruct them. Their empathy is strengthened by their fearlessness to see the truth and trust in a higher purpose in any situation. They take action and move forward leaving no time or space for energy to linger that is not helpful. The empathy Imperial Topazes experience is more global, encompassing an area or a situation rather than an individual. Crystals experience empathy on the individual level. Imperial Topazes also experience empathy for individuals but it is taken in as information and is not personalized like it can be for Crystals.

SELF AWARENESS = GROUP EVOLUTION

Imperial Topazes are not immune to the effects of abuse or injustice; in fact they experience it empathically and totally. But they have a powerful ability to push through fear and past oppressors to the point that they are stronger and wiser because of the hardship. Imperial Topazes are often the first to confront adversity, no matter how difficult, awkward or unorthodox.

Imperial Topazes see all trials as part of a beautiful, intricate design to evolve the human soul. With that perspective they are willing to experience all things life presents—deliberately and all the way through—until complete resolution.

Imperial Topazes are seeking the personal growth that lies at the heart of any difficulty. They can see every situation as something to ride through, including its repercussions, and love finding ways to encourage all to repent, forgive, evolve and move on.

> *"We can't go over.
> We can't go under it…
> We've got to go through it!"*
> From *We're Going on a Bear Hunt*, By Michael Rosen

One of the reasons Imperial Topazes welcome life's injustices and their own imperfections is because they see hardships as a way to fully experience forgiveness and repentance. Their intention is self-awareness and collective awareness in the name of personal and group evolution.

ABUNDANCE & SELF-ACTUALIZATION

Because of this deep acceptance of the process of life, Imperial Topazes have a unique opportunity to effect considerable change in the world. When poverty of mind, body or spirit are present people necessarily focus on finding respite. Humanity seems to operate on a continuum of poverty to abundance—the more comfort people enjoy, the less they focus on lack and the more room they have to focus on adding to humanity. From outside appearances this seems to be true, but Imperial Topazes recognize the real truth, that lack is just a belief and once that belief is shattered, abundance is all that remains no matter what external appearances show.

Instead of being trapped with worry about their circumstances, Imperial Topazes go forward with their purposes, refusing to be hindered. They still have roadblocks on their paths and stewardships over their personal lives and material circumstances, but those things do not hold power over them. They are simply viewed as part of their purposes.

Imperial Topazes realize that nothing external can take away the abundance they feel within themselves. In a scarred, burned landscape, they always know the buds of spring are just about to break through the ashes. This is why their focused, determined, steady countenances are always laced with joy and hope.

PURPOSEFUL
Imperial Topazes are the Aura Personalities most willing to accept and embrace this mortal experience. They understand why they are here, why they have bodies, their stewardships to themselves, others and the world, and are thus able to take full advantage of every opportunity, not in a greedy way, but in a gracious one. Imperial-Topazes are simply wide-awake to all that is available, aware that everything is at their disposal for learning, growth and even enjoyment.

Imperial Topazes are very happy to be alive and are deeply connected and committed to the experience, on every level—mental, emotional, social, physical and spiritual. Part of their mission here is to unveil the possibility of a fully actualized life to the rest of us, primarily by example.

> *"The millions are awake enough for physical labor, but only one in a million is awake enough for intellectual exertion, only one in a hundred millions to a poetic or divine life."*
> From *Walden*, By Henry David Thoreau

MARRIAGE OF OPPOSITES
Imperial Topazes are role models of integration. Opposites find union within them. They are the marriage of yin and yang, winter and spring, decay and rebirth, integrating body and spirit, heart and mind. They do not pedestal or condemn people for any extremes; instead

they respect the processes of life and honor and encourage others on the journey between extremes.

Imperial Topazes are warm and gentle, but also strong and stable. They are accessible, comforting and unassuming, but also confident, direct and stalwart. Their potential is full humility with a backdrop of complete fearlessness.

BALANCE
Imbalance is the thing Imperial Topazes are the most sensitive to in others, but also in themselves. In fact, when they feel out-of-balance, it is all they can focus on. Other people keep going through the motions of life, Imperial Topazes cannot. They will address the imbalance, however long it takes, no matter what is interrupted. They believe it is their biggest responsibility to self and humanity.

Imperial Topazes watch and sense when there is imbalance in their environment or in any human frequency—too electrical, too crowded, too many boundaries, too intellectual, too emotional, too physical, and too energetic. They are drawn to disciplines that encourage environmental and personal awareness and balance, and their preferred schooling revolves around balance as a verb not a noun.

Life throws us out of our natural rhythm quite easily and frequently. Living a balanced life is an active, somewhat messy, and even disruptive process. It means experiencing a lot of imbalance on either end of the spectrum. A goal of balance is not to be confused with one of moderation. Imperial Topazes are not concerned with moderation. Moderate people are controlled people.

Imperial Topazes are concerned with the active dynamic of harmonizing themselves and areas in their lives that are in opposition. They are focused on the opposition, the extremes, the journey between extremes, and the knowledge and growing possible all along the way.

DEMANDING & IMPATIENT
With their full commitment to the journey of life, Imperial Topazes communicate that there is no time to waste, and then they push. They get caught up in the momentum and laser-focused on their purposes.

Imperial Topazes have incredible stamina, but can easily lose balance from their rapid momentum. They get laser-focused on their purposes and have to constantly remember to slow down and pace themselves. Others admire them and like to join them in the journeying, but can sometimes feel pushed beyond their capacities and fall out of their own natural pace. In turn, Imperial Topazes can experience pretty intense agitation when they cannot plough forward because of the agendas and pacing of others; others can feel like irritants or blocks to their forward movement. Of course this is all part of their balancing lessons, and Imperial Topazes are up for the challenge and feel gratitude that others are willing to let them practice with them.

GATHERERS
Imperial Topazes are natural leaders but just like Violets they are not natural managers. It is better for them to forge ahead and let others learn and profit in their wake.

Imperial Topazes have to teach; it just extends from their own rapids lessons in balanced living and processing the cycles of growth to completion. In living and expressing deliberately and purposefully, Imperial Topazes seem to naturally provide environments for people to gather for personal growth.

People cluster around Imperial Topazes because they feel fully accepted by them and want to learn by observing and experiencing them. Imperial Topazes have the feel of both the mother and father archetype in that they simultaneously provide nurturance while stimulating independence and autonomy. They amplify courage and integrity in others and motivate them to live purposefully.

NEW KIND OF RELATIONSHIP
Others get confused in personal relationships with Imperial Topazes, however. This is because Imperial Topazes are modeling a new kind of relationship where each party is fully responsible for themselves. The focus is on self-awareness and personal integrity. There is a learning curve for both parties as they enter such relationships, but the potential for harmony is worth the effort.

WITHOUT REGRET
Despite the messiness of life and the mistakes they inevitably make, Imperial Topazes have high moral intentions in all they do. This does not mean they do not offend or that they do not experience regret; it is just that they are so fully committed to seeing things through to the necessary conclusion, to the best benefit of all involved that there is hardly time or space for regret.

LESSONS IN HYPER-SPEED
Imperial Topazes have all cylinders firing to embrace and push through a personal trial or shortcoming and then

suddenly burst through to its culmination and conclusion, knowledge and intuition rushing in to take its place. The more they move into this rhythm the faster the secession of lessons. Once they embrace this cycle, Imperial Topazes are in heaven because the process that catalyzes growth is their ideal learning environment.

> "...(T)he person of character does not need
> the situation to generate his courage.
> It is a part of his being and a
> standard approach to all life's challenges."
> Michael S. Josephson

Imperial Topazes rapidly vault up, out and through lessons because of their willingness to face them and experience them completely. There is no empty heart for them, no fear of what is on the other side of seeing the truth about themselves. What is there is love from heaven, support from those around them on both sides of the veil, and an incredible energetic momentum that carries them right into their next lessons because of their unshakable belief in all of the above.

> "When you want something,
> all the universe conspires
> in helping you to achieve it."
> From The Alchemist, By Paolo Coelho

~

AURA PERSONALITIES

SHIFTING AURAS

~

AURA PERSONALITIES

CAN THE AURA PERSONALITY CHANGE?
The truth is, I do not know how or why Aura Personalities change or shift. The jury is still out about all the details but they did conclude that shifts happen. Your Main Aura Personality and all of your aura layers can change. Although the Main Aura Personality does not shift very often, there seems to be at least one shift for many people during their lifetime. That said I have seen the Main Aura Personalities of over forty people shift since the first edition of this book was published just a few months ago, and that is just within my small realm of acquaintances.

GLOBAL ENERGY SHIFT
Most of the shifting I have seen began in September of 2012. It is an ongoing phenomenon happening to millions around the world, and it is gaining momentum.

As of yet I do not see any set patterns with shifting except that people are only shifting into Spiritual colors and not into anything else. The forty or so shifts that I know of personally have all shifted into Spiritual Aura colors, either from one Spiritual Aura color to another, or from any of the other Aura Family colors into a Spiritual Aura Family color.

I do not know how shifting works. Are people attracting particular light it into their auric fields, or is the light created by previous choices? Maybe there are other possible explanations as to how people shift and even how we accumulate auric light in the first place, but the thing to note is that a global energy shift is happening.

SOME ARE SHIFTING, OTHERS ARE NOT
That your Main Aura Personality color did not change means nothing about how evolved you are or that you are lacking in any way. If you have not shifted it likely means that your Main Aura Personality, with its attending strengths and opportunities for growth, are what you and those around you need right now.

I recently met a Blue-Amber young man who fully lives in his Aura. He leads a scheduled, predictable life but then stays open to what his heart tells him moment to moment, true to a Blue-Amber.

Blue-Ambers plough forward with goals and tasks like Ambers, but if someone needs their help, they drop their agenda and serve. Then a day comes when Blue-Ambers realize they want to spend all of their time serving others, not just part of it. On that day, they step fully into the gifts of their Aura. They stop worrying about accommodating; they stop caring what other people think; and they get to work serving. They don't waste a minute and everything in their life opens up to support their chosen life of Service.

This moment, when people fully open up to their energy for the first time, is pivotal. Suddenly their game-face is on and nothing can stop them as they blast through the gates. Once that happens, it is over. There is no turning back. They have taken self-awareness seriously enough that it has become self-integrity: True to self no matter what, true to their light no matter what.

One of the greatest joys for me is to see and feel someone fully living true to their Main Aura Personality. It just feels right and solid and clear. In fact, someone taking full-charge of their traits, owning them and using them to the max, is beautiful and empowering to everyone. They accept themselves and embrace all parts of themselves, including their weaknesses. It is not that they have conquered all weaknesses, but that they have fully embraced their strengths to the point that weaknesses just fall to the background. It is a final acceptance and openness to just BE and DO what you ARE without restraint (it feels so liberating even just writing about it!).

FULL EMBODIMENT = COMPLETION
There is a feeling of wholeness and a sense of completion when you experience someone embodying their Main Aura Personality. They have fulfilled, fully owned, integrated, and become the energy of it and, with that completion, they are probably about to shift into a new Main Aura Personality.

Like a star, giving its final light show before it dies out, so it is with Aura Personalities. When you have fulfilled your commitment to the energy of that particular light, it explodes in brilliance and then a new light is born to take its place. This other specific light will integrate with your body and provide you with the particular challenges and abilities that you need next to further progress and shine and serve.

The Blue-Amber mentioned earlier is already embracing who he is far more than most Blue-Amber men of his age. Therefore, more likely than not, a shift is coming for him. I can speculate that Amethyst-Crystal will become his Main Aura Personality since it is his Overlay, but who am I to say? Maybe his Blue-Amber service is needed more than anything else for him and others at this time. Maybe Amethyst-Crystal is just there in support of his Blue-Amber duties. Maybe he will shift into another Spiritual color in his lifetime; maybe he won't.

Maybe we are not all supposed to shift into Spiritual Aura Personalities. Maybe that is not the purpose for everyone and only the role of some for certain periods of time. I suspect our real purpose is to fulfill our unique individual purposes.

> *"Your purpose in life*
> *is to find your purpose*
> *and give your whole heart*
> *and soul to it."*
> Siddhartha Gautama

STRIVING VS. SURRENDERING

I have met many people in the past that mistakenly believed their Main Aura Personalities were Spiritual. At the time I could not understand why they did not own the obvious truth about themselves. The muscle-test was clear and the energy was clear, but there was another thing to consider. Shifting. Some of those people may have been shifting into Spiritual Aura Personalities and were identifying more with what they were becoming than what they had been.

I do not know if shifting is something to strive toward, but I do know that some people complete their missions with their Main Aura Personalities and then shift into Spiritual Aura Personalities. I also know that some people die with Main Aura Personalities that are not in the Spiritual Aura Family and that they have fully completed their missions on this earth and have bestowed upon humanity priceless gifts of love, charity and knowledge. So having a Main Aura Personality that is in the Spiritual Family is not the way for all of us to achieve our life missions.

Striving of itself is not going to shift anyone, nor is worrying about whether or not you have shifted or whether you are supposed to shift. Embracing, allowing, letting go, releasing, accepting, owning, forgiving and surrendering: those are the verbs to think of if you believe you are supposed to shift, or if you are already heading into one. In fact, those verbs are for anyone desiring progression for their soul.

MY EXPERIENCING WITH SHIFTING

For me, active shifting was chaotic and took at least months if not years, but the final shift happened in one very spiritually healing moment. Keep in mind as I describe it here that I had no idea I was going through an energetic shift in my core personality. I only have the privilege of knowing that in retrospect now that I know that shifting happens.

The ongoing process of shifting was like an emotional and energetic rollercoaster ride, but not the fun kind;

more like the creaky, tin can kind in a nightmare where you look down and realize there are no tracks, no other people, no controls of any kind, and you are heading straight for a dark abyss off the edge of a rocky landslide. Shifting from one Main Aura Personality to another felt like extreme soul stretching—a true identity crisis in which there was no way of knowing when, or if, it would end.

My shifting pushed me into an ongoing discussion with God about hidden parts of my personality that I would have preferred to but no longer could keep hidden. It was like the door swung open and all of my unaddressed weaknesses just blasted into clear view, ready to be acknowledged as fast as I was able. They seemed to say, "I've waited long enough. It is time for you to see this part of yourself." And so I did. But interesting to note, this didn't mean I fixed them; I simply acknowledged my weaknesses wholly and truthfully to myself and to God.

Another side effect of shifting was feeling like I was figuratively upside down. All I thought I knew about experiencing life, others, and myself was suddenly no longer known. The accompanying feelings included dips of depression and malaise, tears mixed with elation and chakras over-firing. My energy in so many areas of my body and my life was jumping all over the place from being highly charged to going completely flat.

On a positive note, the speed with which I was learning through shifting was exhilarating. Once I stopped judging the erratic intensity of my emotions, reactions and behaviors and let myself just experience the seemingly never-ending rocket-ship ride that was my new existence, I actually began to enjoy it.

OBSERVING THE SHIFT

These days I see people shifting out of their Main Aura Personalities and into new ones often. After watching so many in such a brief period, I can spot the bewildered look on someone's face and immediately note the feel of their energy when they are shifting. They look like deer caught in the headlights. They feel like someone surrendered, or at a loss, like they have a question on their tongue but are unsure what it is or how to ask it. It is quite funny to observe and, knowing what they are probably experiencing, I nod my head and ask if I can test their aura, and hopefully offer some support or encouragement.

Like many others who have shifted, just previously I had come into complete acceptance of who I was, had compassion for myself in my weaknesses, and joy in giving from my strengths. I had really learned to feel gratitude and love for my Main Aura Personality, and being true to that light had become nearly effortless. That experience of complete self-acceptance seems to be a notable signpost that you are heading into an energetic personality shift.

ENERGY IS THE LANGUAGE FOR THE SPIRITUAL AURA FAMILY

For those that have shifted into Spiritual Family colors that were not just previously, the thing to recognize is that the way you will process life now is via energy; your work will now center on energy. The Spiritual Aura Family is also called the Energy Family—spirit, energy, light are one-in-the-same in this context. You have a new responsibility to energy, it will become your first language, and most of your lessons will be derived from the unseen energy realm and integrated with the tangible realm through you.

LIGHT AS THE SOURCE, THE PATHWAY, THE PASSAGEWAY & THE DESTINATION

As Beings of light, we all probably have Spiritual Family foundations in our auric fields; maybe we all have energetic seedlings to eventually emanate the complete spectrum of light.

As we go through different phases of life, different things are needed from us and for us, and shifting seems to aid these various roles. Our personalities, and their changeability, seem to be perfectly suited to our soul growth and progression.

All auras are energy; all are light. There is no greater or lesser light, just different locations on the light spectrum that signify specific characteristics. If anything, all the colors of light combined would be the only thing to call "greater." All light combined connotes true completion, which is what many know of God, a Being of bright white light beyond comparison, with names in scripture like *Endless, Eternal,* and *Light of the World.*

Whatever auras are—these colorful bands of light that surround our physical bodies—there certainly is something to light that cannot be ignored. Light compels us toward it. We cannot resist emanating it, to whatever degree or combination that we have it. Light seems to be not only fullness but also the ultimate passageway to birth, death and transformation. We hear of near-death experiences where individuals travel toward bright light, and of people who go within the depths of themselves only to find brilliant light at their cores.

Lost in the thought of it, I am so in love with light, its singleness, its infiniteness, and yet the souls spreading it are by far its most valuable aspect. We are an intricate essential part of an endless light show amongst a star-filled expanse; every one of us knowable, every one of us known by the exquisite light we emanate.

~

AURA PERSONALITY PROFILES

~

_____
(name)

_____ & _____
(Main Aura Personality)   (Overlay Aura Personality)

_____
_____
_____
_____
(Outer Layer Aura Personalities)

~

_____
(name)

_____ & _____
(Main Aura Personality)   (Overlay Aura Personality)

_____
_____
_____
_____
(Outer Layer Aura Personalities)

~

_____
(name)

_____ & _____
(Main Aura Personality)   (Overlay Aura Personality)

_____
_____
_____
_____
(Outer Layer Aura Personalities)

©*Aura Personalities*. All rights reserved. No part of this book may be used or reproduced in any manner.

WWW.AURAPERSONALITIES.COM

AURA PERSONALITY PROFILES

~

_____
(name)
_____ & _____
(Main Aura Personality)   (Overlay Aura Personality)

_____
_____
_____
(Outer Layer Aura Personalities)

~

_____
(name)
_____ & _____
(Main Aura Personality)   (Overlay Aura Personality)

_____
_____
_____
(Outer Layer Aura Personalities)

~

_____
(name)
_____ & _____
(Main Aura Personality)   (Overlay Aura Personality)

_____
_____
_____
(Outer Layer Aura Personalities)

©*Aura Personalities*. All rights reserved. No part of this book may be used or reproduced in any manner.

WWW.AURAPERSONALITIES.COM